MW01136611

ABOUT THE AUTHORS

Annabel Streets is an award-winning writer whose books have been published and translated in over 20 countries. A passionate hiker, photographer and cook, she lives in London with her family.

Susan Saunders cared for her mother through more than a decade of dementia, while raising her family and working full-time as a TV producer. She is also the author of two cookery books and a qualified health coach.

Annabel and Susan founded The Age-Well Project in 2014, blogging their way to improved health and longevity at agewellproject.com

THE
AGE
WELL
PROJECT

Easy Ways to a
Longer, Healthier, Happier Life

Annabel Streets and Susan Saunders

PIATKUS

PIATKUS

First published in Great Britain in 2019 by Piatkus
This paperback edition first published in 2021 by Piatkus

5 7 9 10 8 6 4

Copyright © Annabel Streets and Susan Saunders 2019

The moral right of the authors has been asserted.

All rights reserved.
No part of this publication may be reproduced, stored in
a retrieval system, or transmitted in any form or by any means, without
the prior permission in writing of the publisher, nor be otherwise circulated
in any form of binding or cover other than that in which it is published
and without a similar condition including this condition
being imposed on the subsequent purchaser.

A CIP catalogue record for this book
is available from the British Library.

ISBN 978-0-349-41969-5

Typeset in Sabon by M Rules
Printed and bound in Great Britain by
Clays Ltd, Elcograf S.p.A

Papers used by Piatkus are from well-managed forests
and other responsible sources.

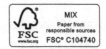

Piatkus
An imprint of
Little, Brown Book Group
Carmelite House
50 Victoria Embankment
London EC4Y 0DZ

An Hachette UK Company
www.hachette.co.uk

www.littlebrown.co.uk

The information given in this book is not intended to replace the
advice given to you by your GP or other health professional. If
you have any concerns about your health, contact the appropriate
health professional. The authors and publisher disclaim any
liability directly or indirectly from the use of material in this
book by any person.

To Richard, Honor and Unity Saunders, whose love inspires me to age well every day; and to Enid Crook, whose dignity and grace in the face of Alzheimer's disease inspired this Project.

Susan

To my parents, Barbara and Peter, who raised me to eat well, walk frequently, read widely and question everything.

Annabel

Contents

Cornerstone Four: Creating The Right Environment For Good Sleep, Lustrous Looks and Enhanced Health

Acknowledgements

This book has been made possible by the efforts, expertise and support of many people. In particular we would like to thank the following researchers and academics for sharing their vast knowledge and giving us invaluable hours of their time: Professor JoAnn Manson and Professor Meir Stampfer of Harvard Medical School; Professor Peter Ellwood of Cardiff University; Professor Carol Brayne of Cambridge University; Professor Michael Hornberger and Professor Anne-Marie Minihane of the University of East Anglia and Norwich Medical School; and Professor John Mathers of Newcastle University.

We'd also like to thank all the researchers, medics and academics whose enlightening lectures we've attended, podcasts we've listened to, and papers we've read – too many to list but we hope you know who you are. Without your dedication and hard work this book would never have been possible.

The nonagenarians we interviewed were both wise and inspiring. Thank you to Sam Almond, Margaret Hibbert, Helen Holder, Douglas Matthews and Lady Kenya Tatton-Brown.

Our early readers provided encouraging and helpful feedback. Thank you Cathy Holmes, Louise Jablonowska, Charlotte Megeney and Janet Tavener. Thank you also to the friends who shared their medical wisdom and personal experiences with us:

you know who you are. And thanks also to Vitória Lucas, for her support and expertise.

We are hugely grateful to our agent, Rachel Mills, who believed in the Project from the beginning (and lit up every meeting with her smile), and also to our editorial team at Piatkus: Anna Steadman, Jillian Stewart, Jan Cutler (for her seamless copyediting), and particularly Zoe Bohm for her calm encouragement. Thanks also to the wider team and to Beth Wright and Aimee Kitson for their help with publicity and marketing.

Many thanks to the loyal readers of our blog, agewellproject. com. Your support, enthusiasm and encouragement have sustained us over the last five years.

But the biggest thanks of all goes to our families, who eat and critique our cooking every day, who hike, run, dance and play ping-pong with us, and who uncomplainingly (mostly) indulge us as we experiment with everything from forest bathing to fasting to fridges bubbling over with kefir. You are the genesis of this book.

Who We Are and How This Book Began

We are two working mothers who met 12 years ago when our daughters were at the same London nursery school. One of us is a TV producer and the other a writer. We both have backgrounds in research and we both have family histories of age-related diseases that struck too soon and too savagely.

Five years ago we stumbled across some research suggesting that we could live longer and better than our ancestors and that our fates weren't determined by the genes of our parents, grandparents and great-grandparents.[1] There was a proviso, of course. The research made it clear that we had to take action in our mid-life years – our forties and fifties. We were both in the latter half of our forties. We just had time. Our Age-Well Project was born.

Both of us grew up in the shadow of disease, watching loved ones die too early from dementia, heart disease and cancer. Or worse, watching them live out their so-called golden years blighted by illness, crippled by arthritis or unable to recognise their own family. One of us had already inherited a chronic disease, and the other was struggling to care for her Alzheimer's-stricken mother. Both of us were raising families, working full-time and paying scant attention to our own health.

Reading that report prompted us to take a good hard look at our lives. We knew our lifestyles were all wrong: irregular eating of the wrong things, sporadic exercise, sleepless nights, chronic stress. After a decade of juggling endless pregnancies and miscarriages, six children and ten elderly parents and in-laws between us, not to mention hugely demanding work commitments, our own health had slipped to the bottom of the pile.

That report also gave us hope, however, making it clear that how we experienced our old age was *our choice*: that we – and nobody else – were responsible for our future health. That small epiphany was like a chink of bright-blue sky on a sluggish grey day.

We started reading more and more: medical books and journals, research reports, culinary histories, tomes on neuroscience. We followed the latest discoveries into ageing. We attended lectures. We spoke to doctors and researchers. We cooked and made time for exercise. And then we blogged. Each week we blogged about a new piece of research and how we were incorporating it into our lives (or not). And each week we posted a recipe to match. For us, blogging was a way of committing to our Age-Well Project, forcing us to stay on the Age-Well wagon while keeping abreast of the hundreds of new developments in geroscience (the science of ageing). Writing a weekly post became a constant reminder that our bodies should be respected, nurtured and treasured. Wading through dense, scientific studies in between day jobs and children wasn't easy, but the support and encouragement of our readers kept us going.

This book explains the most significant changes we made to our everyday lives: there are over 90 short-cuts which research suggests could radically improve our chances of a healthier, happier old age. The results so far? Less stress, better sleep, better behaved guts, defined muscles, more energy, thicker hair, fewer coughs and colds, low blood pressure, consistent weight, and a greater sense of purpose. Will we avoid the diseases of our forebears? We don't know. But we're doing our damnedest. And we feel better than ever.

How to use this book

Each of the changes we made has its own section but is also summarised in an accompanying 'we say' box. We're not suggesting you rush out and make every change. Remember, it's taken us five years and we're still learning. Progression, not perfection, is our motto.

Treat this book like you would a buffet breakfast or a pick 'n' mix salad bar. Start with something you've always wanted to do or something that's easy to incorporate into your daily routine. When you've mastered it, try something else. If it's not working for you, pick a different suggestion. Finding rowing deadly dull? Then try a dance class. Can't get on with lentils? Then try soya beans. Every human body and brain is different – use this book to help find the things that work for you.

We're living in a golden age of medical research. Scientists understand more about the human body than ever before. But any researcher will explain that the more we know the more we realise how *little* we know. Meanwhile, the cures for most diseases of old age remain as elusive as ever. If there's one thing that most medics and scientists currently agree on, it's this: early lifestyle changes have the greatest chance of improving our future. Not a visit to the doctor. Not a pill. Not an operation.

Over and over we were told that many diseases of old age actually begin – silently and stealthily – in middle age. And yet middle age is often the busiest time of our lives. For us, the hardest thing was finding guilt-free time, which is why we focus on the changes offering the greatest result for the least effort: food that takes minutes – not hours – to prepare; activities that are as pleasurable as they're healthy; exercise that's effective in seconds; and family-friendly changes that mean better health for us *and* those we live with.

We also developed little mantras to remind us that time spent on our health was never time wasted. Remember the flight instruction to fit your mask first? Think of your health in the same way and treat your body with the respect it deserves.

A note on understanding research

Perhaps the most significant thing we've learnt over the last half-decade is which reports to heed and which to ignore. A master's degree that included statistics (Annabel) and backgrounds in research (both of us) helped, as did the guidance and advice of our doctor friends and the many experts we've spoken to. This is a vast and unwieldy subject, but we've attempted to use:

- The very latest research (we were updating this book until the last possible minute, to our editor's despair).
- Research carried out on humans (we've included

non-human research only where we felt it was potentially significant).

- Longitudinal studies ideally involving large cohorts over several years.
- Independent research (not funded by an organisation with a vested interest) conducted by reputable, independent institutions and/or individuals.
- Research that's been peer-reviewed and appeared in reputable publications. (We define reputable publications as those included on PubMed.)
- Research that, where possible, reflects the findings of other reports.

There are numerous issues involved in the selection of research – many of which are hugely complex: several reputable publications are heavily funded by external organisations; academia often relies on non-independent funding; careers are made and broken on the back of research; research without a dramatic headline gets little coverage; research that finds 'no results' is left on the shelf ... and so on. We've attempted, within these constraints, to select genuinely credible research done in good faith by acknowledged experts that, in our view, sheds light on a significant aspect of the ageing process.

Finding consensus among the medical community has sometimes proved difficult. In our experience, a moment comes when we *feel* something is right – for us. Perhaps our body responds positively – or negatively – to a change in diet or exercise, or a mode of sleeping or working. Research should never be the tail that wags the dog. When something works for you, let your doctor know and continue with it. If it stops working for you, change it and try something else. Although this book contains many statistics and numbers, always remember that your body is uniquely yours. Learn to listen to it.

Incidentally, it's much easier to listen to a body that is fit, well nourished and (where possible) medication-free. Another reason to nurture yourself.

If you must read the often-contradictory and dramatic headlines, it's worth understanding the terms 'risk' and 'risk factor'. When a headline (or a section in this book!) suggests that your risk could jump by x per cent if you do, or don't, eat/drink/move/sleep, bear in mind that your risk might be very low in the first place. If, for example, your risk of cardiovascular disease is 5 per cent, increasing it by 40 per cent only takes your risk to 7 per cent. To put this further into context, an *average* fit and healthy mid-lifer has a relative heart-disease risk of roughly 3 per cent, meaning that in a group of 100 similarly fit and healthy mid-lifers, three could be expected to have heart disease in the next decade. One's risk level changes over time and is, of course, influenced by many factors, which might typically include whether or not you smoke, your age, weight and lifestyle, for example. To find your possible/approximate risk level, ask your doctor, or cautiously try an online calculator like the QRISK calculator provided by the NHS (http://qrisk.org). Beware: risk calculators are based on algorithms and have been shown to exaggerate risk factors, so use with considerable caution.[2]

Are you still baffled by a newspaper headline? And too time-pressed to check the hard data or run the numbers? We like an NHS website called 'Behind the Headlines' where professionals dismantle and dissect confusing or misleading headlines.[3]

Become your own expert

We're curators of the latest research who tried to find a few answers and incorporated them into our busy lives. We are not – and never have been – doctors, nutritionists, neuroscientists or physiologists. Always consult your doctor or an expert when in doubt. But don't be afraid to ask questions. We urge you to question newspaper articles, research reports, your doctor, this book. Not only because a series of pertinent questions is more likely to find an answer that's right for you, but also because a curious, enquiring mind keeps your brain firing and your cognitive reserves growing.

Lastly, but most importantly: taking responsibility for your health doesn't mean enduring an ascetic life of denial or a guilt-ridden life of angst. We still love a late-night party, a cocktail, a slice of cake, an ice cream, the odd steak and chips. But we view our 'guilty pleasures' as treats to be enjoyed in moderation and entirely without guilt. You have one fleeting, splendid life on this earth. Respect it, but enjoy it.

The Four Cornerstones of healthy ageing

Our research into a happier, healthier old age threw up four areas of our lives that needed addressing: what, when and how we eat and drink; where, when and how we exercise; how best to stay engaged, socially, intellectually and with the right attitude; and how best to manage stress, sleep and the environment surrounding us.

Each area has its ardent advocates: researchers who believe that – be it sleep, diet, exercise or social engagement – their specialism is more important for longevity than anything else. But most scientists now realise how intimately connected each area is. The majority agree that these four facets are inextricably linked, that to disentangle them is difficult and that to elevate one above the others is dangerous. In particular, studies of SuperAgers (a group of elderly people with the cognitive abilities of much younger people) and Blue Zoners (very long-lived people from communities including Okinawa in Japan, the islands of Sardinia in Italy and Ikaria in Greece – now known as Blue Zones)[4] make it clear that we should be improving not only how we eat, but how we move, sleep and behave. We call these our Four Cornerstones of healthy ageing.

The First Cornerstone of healthy ageing: diet

Our Age-Well Project began with food.

You are what – and how – you eat

We read study after study revealing that our ageing bodies and brains benefit from a healthy diet. We devoured every study – metaphorically, of course – before heading to the kitchen, and cooking.

We had to navigate our way, slowly and judiciously. Every diet, from veganism to high-fat-low-carb, has its advocates claiming only their way of eating can deliver a long and healthy life. But, as we sifted through the research, we realised that eating for longevity isn't about fads or extreme diets. It's about balance, moderation and adaptability.

One way of eating cropped up again and again: the

Mediterranean diet. The Mediterranean approach to food bears little resemblance to the refined carbohydrates and processed fats of a typical UK or US diet. The term refers to the food *traditionally* eaten (which is not necessarily the same as the food *currently* eaten) in the communities of Southern Europe: locally grown vegetables and fruits, legumes, grains, olive oil, some fish, small amounts of meat and a little red wine. The diet incudes almost no processed food or refined sugars. Please note that when researchers and doctors talk about a Mediterranean diet they're referring to a traditional, generalised Mediterranean way of eating, which is not what you'd eat on a Spanish holiday, for example.

Early research on the impact of diet on heart disease in the 1950s and 1960s showed that following the Mediterranean diet had a positive effect. More recently, a randomised control trial (the gold-standard of medical research) revealed that a Mediterranean diet, supplemented with olive oil or nuts, reduced the risk of cardiovascular events when compared to a low-fat diet.[5] The diet was also found to improve cognition[6] and reduce the risk of breast cancer.[7]

Every expert we spoke to in the course of writing this book eats a Mediterranean diet. Meir Stampfer, Professor of Medicine at Harvard Medical School, explained, 'There's bona fide, solid clinical evidence to support the benefits of this diet. There's no such evidence to support diets like Paleo or keto. I go where the data is!'.

As we delved deeper we discovered the huge benefits of leafy greens, spices and berries, and the critical importance of vegetables. This doesn't mean being vegetarian or vegan (we're not), but it has meant increasing the number and variety of vegetables on our plates. And with all these plants to eat, it's easier to avoid the foods we don't need: refined carbs, processed meats and sugar.

We've also added plenty of omega-3 fatty acids to our diets, mainly from oily fish and nuts. These essential fatty acids form a critical part of our cell membranes, regulating neurotransmitters (the brain's messaging service), insulin levels and inflammation, leading in turn to fewer heart attacks, and better brain function and gut health.

The role of our microbiota in how we age has been a revelation, with several new studies indicating that our microbiomes might play a more significant role in longevity than previously envisaged. The trillions of microbes populating our gut affect every area of our health, from mental well-being to digestion, responding not only to what we eat, but how and when we eat. We've adopted a version of intermittent fasting (it's not as hard as it sounds!) and increased our fibre intake. Rest assured, cheese, red meat and chocolate are still on the menu. As are beer and red wine. What's not to enjoy?

Key diet principles

- Learn the basics of the Mediterranean diet.
- Focus your diet on vegetables, fruit, whole grains, pulses and fish.
- Remember that olive oil is liquid gold – use it for cooking and salad dressings.
- Add vegetables to every meal. We incorporate them into breakfast, lunch and supper.
- Be good to your gut. Read the sections on microbiota to understand how critically important your microbiome is for your health.
- Cut heavily processed foods from your life: they won't help you age well.

The Second Cornerstone of healthy ageing: exercise

With sedentary careers like ours we knew that more movement was imperative. Reams of research showed that lack of exercise is an important predictor of death from any cause.[8]

Find ways of incorporating movement into your daily life

A study of the Blue Zone nonagenarians of Sardinia attributed their longevity, at least in part, to staying physically active as they aged.[9] This was reflected in a US study of 6,000 women over the age of 60. Their movement – particularly low-intensity physical activity – was measured for two years. The results were clear: the most active women had the lowest risk of dying.[10]

The experts we interviewed were equally clear. JoAnn Manson, Professor of Women's Health at Harvard Medical School, told us, 'The magic bullet for good health is staying physically active. It affects every other factor: blood pressure, insulin sensitivity, blood sugar, cholesterol levels, weight, inflammation levels. Everything is improved by regular physical activity.'

We took up the challenge and added brisk walking to our day. Every day. It's very easy: put on comfortable shoes and head out. Brisk walking has been found to reduce the risk of dying from cardiovascular disease by 24 per cent while increasing cognitive reserve. Walk among trees and you'll also lower blood pressure, blood sugar and heart rate, as well as reducing stress.

When research revealed that sedentary women who fidgeted a lot had no greater risk of premature mortality than very active women, we quickly learnt to fidget. Now we stretch at our desks, keep weights by the kettle and stand up when talking on the phone. We found ways to include more movement in the time we spend with our families: walking our dogs, playing ping-pong, and dancing in the kitchen.

We also added HIIT (high-intensity interval training) to our routines. Despite its uninviting name, HIIT means nothing more than adding short bursts of intensity to your activity. It works on a treadmill, bike or rowing machine: go a little faster for a few seconds, then allow plenty of time to recover. Repeat. HIIT has been found to increase the activity of mitochondria (the 'batteries' of our cells) as we age, and to improve memory. We also added weights to our routine in order to build muscle and bone. We found time to dance, to row (the best all-round exercise, according to experts) and to practise yoga (for strength and mental clarity).

Key exercise principles

- Work movement into your life, every hour and every day. It doesn't have to be power yoga or ballroom dancing. A stretch at your desk or a walk to the corner shop can make a difference.
- Keep weights by the kettle, walk to the station, dust down your bike – think about how you can introduce exercise into your daily life.
- Plan a variety of exercise: a walk one day, dancing with friends the next, a weights workout later in the week.
- Exercise in nature. Walking in the woods or lifting weights in the garden is more beneficial than the same exercise done indoors.
- Consider your constantly evolving bones. Exercise helps keep them strong.
- Always consult your GP when starting a new routine, and stop if it feels too much.

The Third Cornerstone of healthy ageing: staying engaged

Most studies of long-term health have found social interaction and continued mental engagement to be a key predictor of how well we age.

Stay engaged: socialise, think, learn, join in ...

According to neurologist and SuperAger researcher Emily Rogalski, the very healthy elderly have unique personality profiles, which include high levels of resilience, optimism and perseverance. But they also have active, engaged lives involving plenty of stimulating social relationships, and brains continuously challenged by reading, travel, hobbies and learning.

Blue Zoners – the five clusters of exceptionally long-lived people from Okinawa (Japan), Sardinia, Ikaria (Greece), Nicoya (Costa Rica) and Loma Linda in California – are similarly engaged with brain-testing activities and with their communities. Dan Buettner, the original Blue Zone researcher, identified close social and familial bonds as an essential factor in longevity, along with a strong sense of purpose and faith, and a propensity to continue working for as long as possible.

Claudia Kawas, a geriatric neurologist at the University of California, studies SuperAgers and Blue Zoners. She uncovered several factors that both have in common, including attending weekly religious services, reading, and taking part in physical and non-physical leisure activities with other people.[11] We interviewed several SuperAgers for this book and found them, without exception, to be extraordinarily engaged (see Chapter 14).

As we researched, we kept coming across studies demonstrating the age-enhancing powers of: extensive social networks; a happy marriage; pet ownership; meditation; learning languages and instruments; having strong senses of purpose and gratitude; being optimistic; doing something creative; laughter; and developing an enthusiasm for novelty. All of these, it appeared, could affect how healthy, happy and disease-free our later years might be. Researchers don't fully understand why or how, but they suspect it's because activities and behaviours like these keep our brains working, while simultaneously providing an effective antidote to stress.

Here's the paradox, however: many of us settle down in mid and later life, turning away from activities that are difficult, challenging or just different, and settling into old familiar habits and friendships. Yes, mid-life is an excellent time to eradicate chronic stress from our lives. But we need the fizz and buzz of change and novelty to keep us engaged, to keep our brains re-wiring. We need to be getting up and out, not merely for the exercise but for the social interaction it brings.

We've taken the advice of a neuroscientist who's studied the brains of SuperAgers in minute detail, Professor Feldman Barrett.[12] According to Barrett, we should all 'engage in strenuous mental activity on a regular basis ... and dive into it until your brain hurts.'[13] Do this with others to ensure a complete brain and social workout.

Key principles of staying engaged

- Cultivate a wide range of friendships, including new ones.
- Learn something new, and when you've mastered it, try something else. Ideally learn in company rather than

alone. Instruments and languages particularly benefit the brain, but anything that makes your brain ache will do.

- Read books, of all genres. Every day.
- Stay working, paid or unpaid, full-time or part-time.
- Adopt a hobby, creative if you can.
- Develop a mind-set that is optimistic, grateful and purposeful.
- Care for someone: a partner, a dog, those in the local hospice. Someone needs you, and science suggests you might benefit too.
- For maximum bang for buck, select activities that involve other people, a brain workout and movement in a single shot. Dancing, tennis, a walking book group or singing in a choir are excellent options.

The Fourth Cornerstone of healthy ageing: creating the right environment for good sleep, lustrous looks and enhanced health

Getting enough quality sleep has repeatedly been found to help us age better, both physically and cognitively. When we're well-rested, we're also able to enjoy a more robust social life, not to mention feeling more optimistic and empowered. Looking good can help us feel better too, as can toxin-free air, a full set of pain-free teeth, eyes as sharp as pins and a vigorous immune system. While our Fourth Cornerstone focuses on sleep we also investigate several other factors critical to ageing well, from the medications that might be hindering rather than helping us, to vitamin supplements, hidden pesticides and healthier hair.

Master the art of sleep (but don't fret over sleep deprivation)

When we started our careers, sleep was frowned upon. In the heady days of the upwardly mobile 1990s, and beyond into the dot.com era of boom and bust, we worked long days and slept short nights. Sometimes we didn't sleep at all.

The emergence of new technology (laptops, email, social media) and, for us, the arrival of babies, meant sleep became yet more elusive. Suddenly we were living in a 24/7 world. Unsurprisingly, this affected many of our generation, and insomnia became a shared and much discussed topic of conversation. Since then, a series of studies has demonstrated the perils of not sleeping enough, and, contrarily, of sleeping too much.

Poor sleep has now been linked to many degenerative diseases. In 2007 the WHO categorised night shift work as a carcinogen due to its suspected impact on sleep. Neuroscientists at the University of California tracked the sleep patterns and memories of older people, hailing sleep as 'the missing piece of the Alzheimer's jigsaw'.[14] Poor sleep, they explained, creates a channel through which beta-amyloid protein attacks the brain's long-term memory. Another report from Florida's Scripps Research Institute found that quality sleep was crucial for maintaining our long-term memory.[15] A report from the University of Moscow linked poor sleep with twice the risk of a heart attack and four times the risk of a stroke, the author describing poor sleep as a 'killer' – right up there with smoking. Other studies have linked continuous poor sleep to obesity, depression, poor immunity, anxiety, and some cancers. Despite the deluge of studies linking poor sleep to disease, however, a new meta-study of data from 37 million people reveals that insomnia doesn't mean an early death.[16] Worse than not getting enough sleep is *worrying* about not getting enough sleep, so please take note of this meta-study and remind yourself of it whenever you're confronted with a headline indicating that not enough sleep leads to certain death.

It's not only too little sleep that can affect our health. A meta-analysis published in the *Journal of the American Heart Association*, found that sleeping more than needed could also reduce longevity, suggesting that longer sleep is possibly more detrimental to heart health than short sleep.[17] As we edited this book, a report from the National Cancer Research Institute linked too much sleep with a 20 per cent increase in breast cancer risk for each hour slept above 7–8 hours.[18] Seven to eight hours, we're told, is the sweet spot for the average person when it comes to sleep. Bear in mind you might not be average!

On a more mundane note, we knew from our own experience that a string of sleepless nights left us *less* inclined to exercise and *more* inclined to reach for sugary carbs. It also left us more susceptible to coughs and colds, bad moods and low energy levels.

Recently, scientists have discovered that many people are genetically predisposed to poor sleep. But does this mean that we have to consign ourselves to a life of sleep deprivation? The answer is no. Prolonged, poor sleep can be addressed and cured.

When we realised that we could function surprisingly well with no sleep whatsoever and that bi-phasic sleep (sleeping in two stretches rather than one) was not historically uncommon, we stopped worrying. Knowing we were sleeping more like our ancestors did in the past removed much of the angst that accompanied being awake in the middle of the night. We then tackled our poor sleep by following these key principles, all of which are examined in Chapter 11:

Key sleep principles

- Exercise every day, outdoors if possible.
- Embrace guilt-free afternoon naps.
- Change how and what you eat and drink in the evening.
- Allow time to unwind before bed.
- Invest in a new mattress and pillow (if need be) and some essential oils.
- Turn off sources of blue light an hour before you want to sleep.
- Allow fresh air into your bedroom and keep the temperature down.
- Keep regular hours.
- Make time for seven to eight hours of sleep, but don't fret if sleep eludes you. Instead get up or read a book.

Our Fourth Cornerstone also examines other elements within our environment that can affect us as we age. Researchers are becoming increasingly aware of the detrimental impact of industrial chemicals, pollution, even the chemicals within some daily medications. Many of these chemicals are new, making our generation the first to have sustained long-term exposure. To help our bodies survive this onslaught, we need to know what to avoid and what the alternatives are. We also need robust, vigorous immune systems. Our Fourth Cornerstone considers how best to build immunity.

In a highly commercial world, we must also be capable of navigating the marketing promises that assault us daily. Are supplements helpful or harmful? Which, if any, should we invest in? And at what dosage? Similar questions can be applied to beauty products: will they really give us glowing skin and thicker hair or should we focus on food, sunscreen and serums that protect against pollution?

Recent research has thrown the spotlight on healthy teeth and gums – gum disease has been implicated in Alzheimer's – so how should we take care of our mouths? In the meantime, failing eyesight is one of the factors identified as particularly distressing for older people. So how can we start protecting our eyes before it's too late?

Environmental principles for ageing well

- Pay special attention to your gums and teeth.
- Build immunity.
- Know the medications linked, by researchers, to Alzheimer's.
- Eat the right foods for your skin, eyes and hair.
- Use an anti-pollution serum every day and sunscreen when the sun's out.
- Avoid chemical-laden personal care products – opt for organic where possible.
- Forget supplements, except Vitamin D – and zinc for immunity.
- Care for your eyes with regular check-ups.
- Avoid pollution-heavy areas.
- Counter pollution with the right food, the right house plants and an air purifier.
- Avoid pesticides and other chemicals when gardening, eating and cleaning.

CHAPTER 1

The Ageing Body

To understand how we can age better, we need to have a basic grasp of what causes the most prevalent diseases of ageing. Entire books have been written on this vastly complex subject, but we've selected the theories that are currently the most popular with longevity researchers.

How the body ages: the current theories of ageing

Theories of how we age have changed over time, with researchers discarding some and embracing others. The theories not yet eliminated are still being tested in an attempt to understand fully the biological mechanisms that affect how we grow old. We still don't know whether ageing is the result of several different mechanisms operating simultaneously or merely one or two operating independently. But, at the time of writing, the most plausible theories include:

The cross-linking/glycation theory of ageing

As we grow older, our proteins, DNA and other critical molecules can mistakenly cross-link to each other, causing the mobility of proteins and other molecules to be compromised. Damaged proteins are normally broken down and removed by enzymes called proteases, but cross-links inhibit proteases so that the old damaged proteins hang around and cause problems. Cross-linking is thought to be the result of glycation, a process in which glucose molecules stick to proteins causing them to morph into sticky brown molecules called advanced glycosylation end-products (AGEs, funnily enough). These stick to other proteins, effectively disabling them. This process is responsible for wrinkles and cataracts, but some geroscientists now think that it might be responsible for creating the beta-amyloid found in the brains of those with Alzheimer's, as well as possibly playing a role in other diseases of old age.

The free-radical theory of ageing

Free radicals are a toxic by-product of regular cell metabolism that are normally cleared away by antioxidants.[1] If this doesn't happen, they build up causing damage to, and cross-linking between, proteins, DNA and mitochondria (the little powerhouses in our cells). This is known as oxidative damage, and some geroscientists believe it causes diseases such as cancer, cardiovascular disease and Alzheimer's. To add to the burden, our mitochondria's ability to repair DNA damage declines with age for reasons we don't yet understand. However, some scientists think that this ageing of our mitochondria might also contribute to ageing diseases.

The genome maintenance (and the mitochondrial) theory of ageing

As our DNA becomes damaged (through wear and tear, from free radicals or as a result of environmental factors), cell mutations accumulate causing cells to die. The same process takes place in the mitochondria, aggravated by the build-up of free radicals. Humans are effective repairers of DNA, but if we can't keep repairing our DNA, this adds to the debris accumulating in our bodies.

One of the most interesting theories of ageing is the telomere theory of ageing, which has its own section below.

The good news is that most theories of ageing include plenty of scope for us to control how we grow old. All of them point, broadly, in the same direction. Our ability to age well can be enhanced: by eating the right foods, but eating less; taking regular exercise; avoiding stress; and avoiding or countering environmental toxins. Boost these with staying socially and intellectually engaged and our chances of ageing well are dramatically improved.

Ageing and telomeres – their role in your lifespan

Telomeres – a structure at the end of a chromosome – were discovered less than 50 years ago by a trio of scientists who later won a Nobel prize for their work. A popular theory of ageing now speculates that the length of our telomeres determines our lifespan; in other words, the longer our telomeres, the greater our chances of a long and healthy life. Meanwhile, shortened telomeres are considered a 'hallmark of ageing'.

Telomeres sit on the ends of our chromosomes like the protective tips of shoelaces. As we age, our telomeres become shorter, causing cells to stop functioning properly and eventually to die. Fortunately, our cells produce an enzyme called telomerase, which enables cells to continue dividing and allows telomeres to be preserved, and even replenished. Some scientists now believe that producing telomerase might be more important to our health and longevity than having long telomeres; however, as we age, our bodies also produce less telomerase.

Either way, shorter telomeres have been linked to wrinkles, cognitive impairment, Alzheimer's disease, lung disease, heart disease and a smaller hippocampus (the part of the brain associated with memory), among other things. Scientists, however, have a clear picture of what our telomeres like and don't like, and the factors hindering the efficient production of telomerase. Environmental and lifestyle factors seem to have a significant impact: stress, inflammation, smoking, high alcohol consumption, obesity, lack of exercise, pollution, poor diet, and pessimism – all affect our telomeres.

Many observational studies have linked longer telomeres with a plant-rich Mediterranean diet. Research shows that people living in the Mediterranean have longer telomeres,[2] and the more rigorously they hold to a Mediterranean diet, the longer their telomeres become – whereas shorter telomeres have been linked to sugary drinks and processed food/meat products.[3]

Research in ageing rats shows that telomere length is preserved when protein is restricted. Reflecting this, a recent study in the *Journal of Gerontology* suggests that what telomeres really appreciate is a low-protein, high carbohydrate diet.[4] In this study, fat consumption had little effect, but the telomeres also responded to vitamins C, D, E, folate and beta-carotene, zinc and magnesium, all of which protect against oxidative stress and inflammation, which in turn protect the length of our telomeres. Telomeres also respond to polyphenols, as found in a study of elderly Chinese tea-drinkers whose telomeres were the equivalent of five-years longer than those of non-tea drinkers. Indeed, antioxidant-rich food appears to lengthen telomeres, with researchers highlighting the following as being of particular benefit: seeds, nuts, legumes, seaweed and coffee. In women, a diet high in wholegrain fibre also meant longer telomeres.

Many other factors affect both the length of our telomeres and our capacity to produce telomerase, from our genes to how we were raised. But the work of Professors Blackburn and Epel (among others) shows how we can actively strengthen and lengthen our telomeres and supercharge our telomerase, in order to improve our healthspan.* Their work identifies several simple things that we can do to take charge of how well we age. We'll paraphrase some of it here, but we urge you to read their book for a fuller explanation.[5]

Stress is hugely detrimental to telomeres. Meditation, mindfulness and qigong have been shown to preserve telomeres better, with one study finding that regular meditators achieved a 43 per cent increase in telomerase,[6] a finding repeated in other meditation studies.[7]

The advice of Professors Blackburn and Epel is to follow a Mediterranean diet, with plenty of the telomere-loving ingredients listed above, and plenty of omega-3 fats. New research

---

* Note: Because telomerase (and very long telomeres) has been linked to cell replication, it might be implicated in cancer. For this reason experts don't recommend that telomerase is boosted artificially using supplements. A healthier lifestyle is quite adequate.

shows that people with higher concentrations of omega-3 in their blood have longer telomeres. Blackburn and Epel say that omega-3 consumption should be a 'priority', ideally through diet rather than supplementation.

Bear in mind that changing the length of your telomeres or improving your telomerase production can take months, if not years, so start slowly, making incremental and sustainable changes to your lifestyle. We started by increasing our daily exercise and stockpiling tinned sardines, which we now eat once a week.

Look after your telomeres: we say

- Avoid sweetened drinks and processed meat.
- Consume omega-3s (found in oily fish).
- Drink coffee.[8]
- Consider intermittent fasting or time-restricted eating (see Chapter 3). Caloric restriction in mice has been associated with longer telomeres.[9]
- Develop positive, resilient thinking.[10]
- Exercise for 30 minutes a day.[11]
- Get at least seven hours of quality sleep a night.[12]
- Rise and sleep at the same time each day.[13]
- Avoid pesticides.[14]
- Watch out for PAHs (polycyclic aromatic hydrocarbons), found in barbequed meats, cigarette smoke and exhaust fumes.[15]
- Live somewhere that makes you happy; enjoy nature and nurture your social network.[16]

The role of your microbiome for good health

One of the biggest recent breakthroughs in human science has been our understanding of the microbiome: the vast throbbing universe of bacteria (and a few fungi, viruses and protozoa) that live on and in us. Our microbial cells outnumber our human cells by ten to one, and most of them live in our colon and small intestine. From here, they regulate many aspects of our well-being: they kill off harmful bacteria; they help synthesise vitamins; they stimulate our immune systems; they regulate our body weight.

Studies of the faecal remains of our ancestors and of hunter–gatherer tribes such as the Tanzanian Hadza[17] show how sparse the modern Western microbiome has become, leading scientists to speculate about a link between depleted microbes and many of the diseases that plague us, from obesity to type-2 diabetes to dementia, Alzheimer's, Parkinson's, osteoporosis and rheumatoid arthritis.[18]

As we age, our microbes become more and more depleted. Indeed, early research suggests that how we age might be determined by the quality and quantity of our microbiome. We need to pay particular attention to our microbiomes in mid-life: studies show that our gut bacteria alters with age, often becoming sparser and less diverse. Scientists speculate that this reduction in diversity could play a role in the inflammatory and neurodegenerative diseases of old age. It's not all doom and gloom, however: recent studies of exceptionally long-lived people in Italy and China found their microbiomes richer and more diverse than those of their younger counterparts,[19] leading the authors of one report to conclude that a diverse microbiome could be a precursor to healthy old age.

If you really want to know what's happening in your

microbiome, you could do as we did: a faecal (poo) analysis. It's a simple, painless exercise that involves ordering a kit from British Gut, American Gut or uBiome (all not-for-profit organisations), then a quick swab, which is posted in a sealed envelope. And, finally, a long wait. The results show exactly what's living in your colon, comparing it to the average microbiome. If you use British or American Gut, you also see (weirdly) how your microbiome compares to that of food writer Michael Pollan.

The good news is that your microbiota can be improved quickly and easily. A seminal study in *Nature* magazine compared the gut microbiomes of people eating an entirely animal-based diet (meats, cheeses and eggs) with one that was completely plant-based (grains, legumes, vegetables and fruits). Just one day on either diet was enough to shift the gut microbiome of participants dramatically.

The best way to start caring for your microbiome is to feed it lots of the prebiotic-rich food it loves. That's not the *pro*biotics that introduce bacteria into your gut (we'll come to those in the next chapter), but the fibrous food that nourish the bacteria already living inside you – and that will feed any new bacteria you introduce via fermented food.

Prebiotics alone have been able to improve gut microbiota dramatically. A study reported in the *British Journal of Nutrition* showed that the consumption of prebiotics produced a very positive effect on both gut microbiota and the immune systems of 40 volunteers aged 65–80. Meanwhile, a recent study found that introducing a prebiotic-rich ingredient into the diet of obese, osteoarthritic mice, entirely reversed the symptoms of their osteoarthritis.[20]

A diverse microbiome requires a diverse diet, as highlighted by the first results from the American Gut Project, which found that people with the broadest plant-based diets had the most bacterially diverse microbiomes.[21] In particular, those eating more than 30 different types of plant each week had far greater diversity than those consuming 10 or fewer plants per week. Scientist, Jeff Leach, founder of both The Human Food Project and American Gut, advocates eating as many different plant varieties each week as possible, but top of his list is the humble leek due to its very high fibre content. Jeff eats a lightly cooked leek every day.

Other foods with exceptionally high prebiotic content include: Jerusalem artichokes, onions and garlic, dandelion leaves, bananas (the greener the better), asparagus, apples (Granny Smiths are particularly rich in prebiotics), oats (ideally uncooked), broccoli stalks, pulses, and whole grains.

Combine a prebiotic-rich diet with probiotic-rich food (like yoghurt) and, as Edmond Huang, a metabolic biologist at the University of California, says you might begin to see improvements in a matter of days or weeks.[22] Yes, it's that dramatic.

Your microbiome: we say

- Invest in a faecal analysis, if you're interested or concerned. You'll also be helping the scientific community improve its knowledge of the microbiome.
- Increase the amount of prebiotic-rich food in your diet (we aim for 30 different plants a week) and try to eat something with a high prebiotic content every day.
- Eat the stalks, peel and – if you fancy it – the core. The more fibrous and stringy the fruit or vegetable, the more appealing it will be to your microbiota.

Tackle inflammation

An increased concentration of inflammatory markers in the bloodstream is as much an indication of ageing as crows' feet and laughter lines. Inflammation is so intrinsically linked to ageing that a new term has been coined: 'inflamm-ageing'.[23] Fortunately, there are plenty of ways to keep inflammation at bay.

Inflammation is our friend when we need an acute response to a sting, cut or other injury: it helps us heal. But it's not so useful when it's chronic and long term, which is exactly what happens as we age. Ageing causes the body to behave as if it's under threat, constantly pumping extra proteins into the blood. Doctors refer to this as 'low-grade inflammation', or LGI. It plays a central role in all the chronic conditions of old age, which is why reducing inflammation in mid-life is critical. Insulin resistance (see page 39) and type-2 diabetes, cognitive decline, weight gain, loss of mobility, reduced immunity, cancer and cardiovascular disease are all linked to inflammation. Recent research suggests that inflammation is as vital a target as cholesterol in preventing heart disease.[24]

In addition, LGI is linked to the frailty that often comes with growing older.[25] Frailty results from the cumulative decline of all our physical functions, making us more vulnerable to internal and external stresses. Higher levels of inflammation have been found in people with reduced handgrip strength, a standard test for frailty.[26]

Why, then, does inflammation happen as we age? There are several possibilities, and it's probably a combination of them all:

- Mitochondrial damage – as our telomeres shorten with age, mitochondrial DNA finds its way into our bloodstream, triggering inflammation[27] (see the earlier section in this chapter for how to protect our telomeres and mitochondria).

- The failure of autophagy – the 'cleaning up' process that happens in our cells.
- Cell senescence – when cells stop dividing and reproducing.
- Our immune system's increased inability to respond to inflammation as we age.
- An imbalance in gut microbiota.[28] Our microbiome changes as we age, and this is associated with increased inflammation, which in turn impacts our immune system.
- It's possible that inflammatory material makes its way to the brain, where it triggers further inflammation in the hypothalamus, the part of the brain responsible for hunger, sleep and circadian (sleep) rhythms. When that goes awry, further ageing takes place.

Tackling LGI is critical to prevent or delay the onset of almost all degenerative age-related conditions. The good news is that a few simple changes to our diet could make a huge difference.

Low-grade inflammation: we say

- Follow the Mediterranean diet.[29] Research shows that a higher intake of whole grains, vegetables, fruits, nuts and fish is associated with lower inflammation.
- Eat lots of antioxidant-rich foods, such as brightly coloured fruit and vegetables. There's a link between

oxidative stress and inflammation, so antioxidants bring
positive benefits.

- Feed your gut – the healthier and more diverse your
microbiome, the less inflammation you'll have.

- Get plenty of probiotics from fermented foods such as
live yoghurt, kefir and miso. We try to have a little of
something fermented every few days. Some scientists
believe probiotics might have a role to play in reducing
inflammation, although more research is needed.

Keep your waist trim

Obesity rates are at an all-time high. More than two thirds of adults
in the Western world are classified as overweight, and experts think
that our current epidemic of obesity will be one of the biggest deter-
minants of longevity – or mortality – for those of us alive today.

Research consistently shows that obesity in mid-to-late life
increases the risk of dementia[30] as well as increasing our risk of
type-2 diabetes, high blood pressure, arthritis, several cancers,
depression and cardiovascular disease.[31] Let's put it another
way: in our five years of investigations, we've not come across a
single study, report or book suggesting excess body fat in mid-
life is good for us. Nor, as we travelled the country interviewing
nonagenarians and longevity experts, did we once meet anyone
even the tiniest bit overweight.

At the very time we need to slim down, however, we typically
get larger. As we age, our metabolism tends to slow, we begin to
lose muscle and we often become more sedentary.

On our Age-Well Project we tackled our creeping weight in several ways. But first we threw away our bathroom scales. Why? Because it's not how much we weigh that matters, but the amount of abdominal fat we're carrying – sometimes called visceral or active fat or adipose tissue. We put all those body mass index (BMI) calculations aside too. Waist circumference and waist-to-hip ratio (WHR) are the new BMI when it comes to ageing, because of their greater accuracy for measuring abdominal fat, the fat lying deep within our mid-section, wedged between our lungs, heart, liver and intestines. It's this fat that's the most dangerous as we get older.

Studies show that storing fat around our internal organs (which often appears as a pot belly or an apple-shaped body as opposed to a pear-shaped body) increases our risk of cardiovascular disease, diabetes and heart attacks as well as contributing to chronic inflammation, oxidative stress, insulin sensitivity and metabolic health.[32] More recently, studies have indicated that an increase in WHR is often associated with reduced cognitive function.[33]

Anyone can carry abdominal fat – including thin people – but women need to be particularly vigilant. In a study involving 500,000 adults, researchers found that waist circumference was the most accurate predictor for heart attacks, particularly for women. An earlier report found that people with large waists had the same risk of developing diabetes as those categorised as clinically obese. Again, the link was stronger in women. Another report found that waist-to-hip ratio predicted cardiovascular disease better than either BMI or waist circumference.[34]

Measure your waist and your waist-to-hip ratio

Here's how to measure your **waist circumference**: use one hand to locate the top of your hip bone; use your other hand to locate the bottom of your ribcage. The midway point between hipbone and ribcage – usually just above the navel – is where you measure, after removing any clothing and fully exhaling. If you're female, your waist should be no larger than 80cm. If you're male, it should be no larger than 94cm.

Here's how to calculate **your waist-to-hip ratio** (WHR): measure your hips at their widest point (on the skin not on clothing), then divide your waist measurement by your hip measurement. Use the World Health Organization chart below to identify your risk level.

• Health risk	• Men	• Women
• Low	• 0.95 or lower	• 0.80 or lower
• Moderate	• 0.96–1.0	• 0.81–0.85
• High	• 1.0 or higher	• 0.86 or higher

Use these measurements in conjunction with your BMI to get a fuller picture of how your current weight could impact your future health.

Equally, for older people being too thin is as dangerous as being too fat. Claudia Kawas, geriatric neurologist at the

University of California, found that SuperAgers with a very low body mass index after the age of 80 were more likely to die than those with a normal BMI.[35] Being underweight also increases a woman's risk of osteoporosis and anaemia.

Maintaining a healthy weight: we say

- Know your waist circumference and waist-to-hip ratio (WHR).
- Remind yourself that exercise is no longer optional – move more (see Chapter 7), specifically calorie-burning cardio exercise that builds up a sweat. Recent research shows that exercise suppresses appetite, making it doubly effective. It seems that the heat generated by exercise stimulates receptors in the brain that suppress hunger.[36]
- Eat less – smaller portions, not before bed, and fewer snacks (see Chapter 3).
- Eat right – cut out processed food.
- Try periods of fasting – either longer overnight fasts or daily fasts (see Chapter 3).
- Get the right amount of sleep – poor sleep is also associated with weight gain.
- If you're over the age of 80, don't become underweight.

Keep an eye on your blood pressure

High blood pressure is one of the fastest, stealthiest ways to shorten your life.

As we age, our blood pressure often rises, and frequently for no apparent reason. High blood pressure has no symptoms, so we can't tell whether it's dangerously high or safely low: recent statistics suggest one in four of us has high blood pressure without knowing it.

Yet keeping our blood pressure low is one of the most important things we can do to prevent diseases of old age. Spiralling blood pressure has been linked to premature memory loss, stroke, heart failure and heart attacks. It also doubles the risk of Alzheimer's, increases the risk of vascular dementia six-fold and can lead to kidney failure and loss of eyesight.

From around the age of 30, our blood vessels begin to stiffen and narrow, making the heart work even harder (your heart contracts every second to deliver oxygen and nutrients to every corner of your body, a mind-boggling feat that no machine could replicate). This extra work means our hearts grow thicker walls – which results in higher blood pressure. If it becomes too high, doctors call it hypertension. By the age of 65 our risk of developing hypertension is 50 per cent. In other words, half of us will have hypertension. Worryingly, a new report suggests that even slightly raised blood pressure over the age of 50 might be indicative of very early dementia in some individuals.[37]

Diet, exercise and stress are thought to play a role. A diet rich in fruit and vegetables appears to be protective. And yet a recent survey[38] found that high blood pressure was linked to high salt intake irrespective of the 'healthiness' of one's diet, suggesting that a good diet might not be protective if it's heavily salted.

What appears to work, however, is a combination of eating a Mediterranean (or DASH – Dietary Approaches to Stop Hypertension) diet and cutting back on salt. According to one study combining the DASH diet (which is, to all extents and purposes, a Mediterranean-style diet) with additional salt reduction was more effective than taking anti-hypertensive drugs, particularly for those at the highest risk.[39]

Even more intriguing are early findings linking healthy blood pressure levels with the gut. A study reported in *Nature* found that a well-balanced microbiome protected against high blood pressure, although the researchers weren't sure how or why.[40] Another study found that regularly drinking kefir (fermented milk) reduced blood pressure (as well as improving the guts) of rats after only nine weeks.[41]

Meditation has consistently been found to reduce blood pressure, particularly among those with levels that are elevated but not yet high. A Harvard study found that 15 minutes of daily meditation for eight weeks resulted in significant reductions in blood pressure for over half the cohort.[42]

Regular movement is essential for keeping blood pressure down. A recent study found that sitting for only two hours can cause significant jumps in blood pressure.[43]

Last but not least, enjoy regular sunshine. Studies suggest that exposing skin to the sun changes the levels of nitric oxide (NO) in our skin and blood, effectively reducing blood pressure.[44] We spend 20 minutes – without sunblock, but no longer – in the sun whenever we can, weather and temperature permitting.

Blood pressure: we say

- Know your blood pressure and have it tested regularly. You don't need to visit your doctor – the practice nurse at your GP's surgery, some pharmacies and gyms offer blood pressure testing. Home monitors are thought to be accurate too.

- Don't panic after a single high reading. GPs need a series of readings, often from different times of the day, to create a consistent picture.
- Keep an eye on your weight. Obesity contributes to raised blood pressure.
- Keep your salt intake sensible by avoiding processed food.
- Switch to a Mediterranean or DASH diet.
- Do 30 minutes of exercise that makes you sweaty and breathless five times a week. We like dancing, rowing, hill walking and table-tennis. But, more importantly, find something you enjoy.
- Look after your gut by including fibrous and fermented food in your diet.
- If your blood pressure's rising, consider a meditation class or app.
- Never sit for longer than two hours without moving. If you have to sit, try fidgeting.
- Get sun whenever you can.
- As ever, quit smoking, go easy on the alcohol and try to sleep well at night.

Your type-2 diabetes risk

One in 16 people in the UK has diabetes in some form, more than double the number 20 years ago.[45] The vast majority of these have type-2 diabetes, a chronic, lifestyle-related disease.

Although it can be managed with medication, diet and lifestyle changes, type-2 diabetes is the gateway condition to a host of other health problems, including kidney failure, heart disease and dementia. The more we can do to reduce our risk or manage the symptoms, the better.

There are several risk factors (see the box overleaf) for type-2 diabetes but key is the body's failure to respond to insulin, a hormone produced by the pancreas to mop up glucose. When everything is working normally, insulin helps glucose move from the bloodstream to the cells in muscles, fat and liver, where it's used for energy. But if those cells stop responding to insulin, the pancreas produces more insulin to keep glucose out of the bloodstream: a process called insulin resistance. If the pancreas fails to produce enough insulin, blood sugar levels remain high,[46] a condition known as pre-diabetes. It's a risk factor for type-2 diabetes, obesity and heart disease. Increasingly, it's been linked to a higher risk of dementia.

Left untreated, this build-up of glucose in the blood causes ageing by creating AGEs in the body. If ever there was an appropriate acronym, it's AGEs. As we saw earlier, it stands for advanced glycation end-products, by-products of high blood sugar. The excess glucose binds with protein to make an AGE. Once made, they accumulate in our bodies. AGEs are linked to many of the complications of diabetes, including nerve damage, eye problems, kidney disease, hardening of the arteries (atherosclerosis), dementia and erectile dysfunction.

There's now a clear link between dementia and diabetes: Alzheimer's has been called the 'diabetes of the brain' or 'type-3 diabetes'. Numerous studies have shown that people with type-2 diabetes have an increased risk of dementia: it's one of the biggest risk factors for the disease. Researchers think that the hippocampus, the part of the brain linked to memory and learning, can become 'diabetic' in the same way that our liver and fat cells can.[47] Cognitive decline resulting from type-2 diabetes might actually be early stage Alzheimer's.

More terrifying still, high blood sugar impacts the brain in such a way that it precipitates cognitive decline without diabetes being present. A 10-year study of over 5,000 people found that those with high blood sugar had a faster rate of cognitive decline than those with normal blood sugar.[48] This held true even when blood sugar wasn't high enough to trigger diabetes.

The risk factors for diabetes

Diet isn't the only risk factor for diabetes. Other factors include:[49]

- Being overweight: obesity is the biggest type-2 risk.
- A sedentary lifestyle.
- High blood pressure.
- High cholesterol levels.
- Genetic factors – is a family member diabetic?
- Having previously had gestational diabetes.
- Smoking.

The good news is that type-2 diabetes can be entirely reversed with nothing more than lifestyle changes. Low-carb and low-calorie diets have been used to successfully treat diabetes by reducing weight, blood sugar and reliance on medication.

Blood sugar levels and diabetes: we say

- Manage your blood sugar levels and the risk factors as listed in the box opposite. We've overhauled our diets, made exercise a priority and now have our blood pressure checked every few months.
- Don't leave symptoms of type-2 diabetes untreated. It's estimated that over half a million people in the UK, and 175 million worldwide,[50] have undiagnosed diabetes.
- Symptoms can include tiredness, hunger – even after meals; constant thirst; urinating more than usual, particularly at night; blurred vision and itchy skin.
- Worried? Have your blood sugar levels checked – your GP can run a simple test.
- You're looking for a haemoglobin A1c (HbA1c) level of less than 42mmol/mol. Levels of HbA1c of 42–47mmol/mol are considered a high risk of developing type-2 diabetes.[51] Above that indicates possible type-2 diabetes.
- Watch out for foods that cause elevated blood sugar and put pressure on the pancreas to produce insulin: sugary treats, refined carbohydrates, fast food and fizzy drinks are the worst offenders.
- www.diabetes.co.uk runs a low-carb programme. Michael Mosley's *The 8-Week Blood Sugar Diet* is a low-calorie programme for diabetes control.

Cholesterol – a changing hypothesis

Our understanding of cholesterol and its role in our health has advanced hugely in recent years. For our parents' generation cholesterol was just *bad*. We now know that cholesterol is vital for many biochemical processes: helping to produce bile for digestion, balancing hormones, creating vitamin D and lubricating cell membranes.

We've also learnt that much of the cholesterol in our bodies is made by the liver, rather than coming from what we eat. Sources of dietary cholesterol, like eggs, liver and prawns, don't raise blood cholesterol. Rather they prompt our bodies to makes less cholesterol, so that levels generally balance out. Where, then, do high cholesterol levels come from? They're often genetic, but they're also linked to smoking, a lack of exercise, too much alcohol and a diet high in saturated and trans fats and refined carbohydrates.

There are two types of lipoproteins that carry cholesterol in the bloodstream: low-density lipoprotein (LDL) aka the 'bad' cholesterol which forms hard plaques in the arteries, increasing cardiovascular disease risk; and high-density lipoprotein (HDL) – referred to as the 'good' cholesterol which protects against heart disease by clearing the build-up of LDL and transporting it back to the liver where it's re-used or excreted. We want fewer LDL particles in the bloodstream, and more HDL, to reduce heart-attack risk.

Recent research has shown that this analysis of cholesterol can be broken down even further: the size of the particles making up both types of cholesterol is also relevant. They range from small, dense particles, through to large 'fluffy' ones. It's the small particles of LDL that attach themselves to artery walls and raise heart-attack risk. Big fluffy LDL particles are relatively benign.

Similarly, big fluffy particles of HDL are more protective against heart disease, but high levels of small, dense HDL have been linked to higher risk of heart attacks.[52]

A recent study tracked almost 6,000 people with cardiovascular disease for four years and found that those with the lowest and highest levels of HDL were most likely to have a heart attack. The researchers suggested HDL could become dysfunctional when levels are very high, losing its ability to protect the heart.[53]

Triglycerides are a form of fat the body uses for energy. They come either from dietary fat (animal or plant sources) or they're made by the liver after we've eaten. They circulate in the blood until they're either used for fuel or stored as fat. When we consume, or make, too many triglycerides, levels in our blood stream rise. Raised triglyceride levels might contribute to the hardening of the arteries and can be a symptom of pre-diabetes. They often go hand-in-hand with low HDL levels. When you have your cholesterol levels checked, ask for a full lipid profile that covers triglycerides.

We had our cholesterol and triglycerides levels checked (by our GP) as part of our Age-Well Project. Everyone between the ages of 40 and 75 should do this every five years. You're looking for total cholesterol levels of less than 5mmol/L (millimoles per litre). Check out www.heartuk.org.uk for a detailed breakdown.

Cholesterol: we say

- Don't cut out foods high in dietary cholesterol – eggs, full-fat dairy, shellfish, sardines and liver all bring huge health benefits.

- A study revealed that people eating three whole eggs a day had a greater increase in HDL, and decrease in LDL, than those who consumed an equivalent amount of egg substitute.[54]
- Avocados have been shown to have a beneficial effect on total cholesterol, and triglyceride, levels.[55]
- Other cholesterol-lowering foods include pulses, nuts, soya beans, fruit and vegetables.
- Many studies show that exercise has a positive effect on cholesterol levels.

BDNF – fertiliser for your brain

Brain-derived neurotrophic factor (BDNF), a protein found inside the brain, is often described as Miracle-Gro for the mind: essentially it stimulates the growth and survival of brain cells and the synapses that connect them. Having a plentiful supply of BDNF means that you learn more quickly, remember more clearly, and age more slowly. The more BDNF you have, the better your brain works, whereas low levels of BDNF have been linked to cognitive impairment, Alzheimer's, depression and obesity.

As we age, we produce less and less BDNF, however. Luckily, there are plenty of things you can do to boost your BDNF – and most of them can be done easily and safely at home. Indeed, most of them are also bedrocks of our Age-Well programme:

Exercise – vigorously and regularly. Thirty minutes of vigorous exercise a day (at 60–75 per cent of your maximum heart rate), over a few months, can boost production of BDNF.[56]

Look after your microbiome A healthy microbiome, rich in *Lactobacillus* and bifidobacteria, seems to increase BDNF.[57] Include some fermented food in your diet.

Fasting or caloric restriction Intermittent fasting (see page 74) appears to raise BDNF. But like exercising, it's not a quick fix and you'll need to persevere.[58]

Cut sugar and saturated fat People on diets high in refined sugar and saturated fat often have low levels of BDNF. As with exercise and fasting, BDNF responds slowly to a change of diet, so don't expect instant results.[59]

Get enough sunlight BDNF levels react to our exposure to sunlight. A Dutch study found that serum BDNF levels rose and fell according to the availability of sunshine. On moderately sunny days expose as much skin as possible for up to 20 minutes without sunscreen. A recent study found that sunscreen of factor 15 or higher reduces vitamin D production by 99 per cent.[60] Supplement with vitamin D during darker months.[61]

Eat a diet rich in polyphenols, omega-3 fats and turmeric (or consider supplementing with curcumin). Studies in rats suggest both curcumin and omega-3 (specifically DHA found in oily fish) may increase BDNF.

Improve your sleep People suffering from sleep deprivation have been found to have less BDNF, and the worse their insomnia, the lower their levels of BDNF.[62]

Keep an eye on stress Whereas short-term stress can boost BDNF temporarily (as can a single night of poor sleep), chronic stress, like chronic insomnia, depletes it. Studies have found that yoga and meditation, done intensively over three months, can raise production of BDNF.[63]

Keep an eye on your weight Several studies have linked obesity to reduced BDNF, while obese children often become BDNF-deficient adults. This may simply be a symptom of not exercising or consuming too many calories, but research suggests the link might go beyond this.

Boosting BDNF: we say

- Exercise for 30 minutes every single day, without fail. A brisk walk is all it takes.
- Do your best to sleep well and manage stress.
- Eat some form of prebiotic and probiotic most days, along with oily fish at least twice a week, and fruit and vegetables with every meal.
- Undergo the odd fast.
- Get out whenever the sun shines and supplement with vitamin D in the winter months.

Stress and how to beat it

There have been times when we've felt completely overwhelmed by stress. It sapped our strength, robbed us of joy and wrecked our sleep patterns. Juggling high-pressure jobs, elderly parents, young children and the demands of modern life, we fell victim (like so many others) to the constant pressure to do – and have – it all. As part of this Project, we learnt to reduce stress when we could, and to manage it when we couldn't. One of the advantages of ageing, we've found, is that it's easier to put stressful situations into perspective and to focus on the good things in life.

Unsurprisingly, the first study linking stress and ageing focused on mums. In 2004, researchers at the University of California compared a group of mothers looking after children with chronic illness with those caring for healthy children. Those with chronically ill kids aged more quickly. The researchers pointed out that the issue was also one of *perceived* stress – some carers perceived their situation as less stressful than others, and so aged less rapidly.[64]

Why is stress ageing? It comes back to telomeres, those protective caps at the ends of our chromosomes (see page 23). Every time a cell divides, telomeres get shorter. In the ageing process, telomeres eventually get so short that the cells can no longer divide, and they die. In the 2004 Californian study, the mothers with the highest levels of *perceived* stress had telomeres that were around a decade shorter than those of less-stressed women.

Work-related stress has a similar impact. A Finnish study found that participants with the most job stress had the shortest telomeres.[65] Work stress has also been associated with a 50 per cent increased risk of atrial fibrillation, an irregular heartbeat that causes 20–30 per cent of all strokes.[66]

Prolonged exposure to work-related stress has been linked to an increased likelihood of lung, colon, rectal and stomach cancer, and non-Hodgkin lymphoma in men. Again, the highest risk of developing cancer was among the men with perceived high stress levels.[67]

Chronic stress can contribute to the development of Alzheimer's. Swedish researchers found that elevated levels of stress steroids in the brain can inhibit general brain activity. This, in turn, was found to accelerate the development of Alzheimer's in mice. Another rodent study found that in times of stress, a hormone called corticotrophin-releasing factor is created in the brain. This increases the production of amyloid beta, implicated in the formation of the plaques and tangles that may lead to Alzheimer's disease.[68] Middle-aged adults with high levels of the stress hormone cortisol had smaller brain volume and performed less well in memory tests than those with lower levels.[69]

Professor JoAnn Manson of Harvard feels that stress is one of the most critical health issues of our age:

I'm increasingly aware of how important stress reduction is, particularly for women. Stress is a risk factor for heart disease, cognitive decline, diabetes, and maybe even cancer. It's very understudied but we know enough to encourage people to manage stress. We need to be physically active but we also need to aim for positive personal interactions with family and friends. It's important that you're enjoying yourself and not with people who make you feel stressed.

JoAnn manages stress by taking short walks.

Studies suggest that how we respond to daily stress might also affect our cognitive function. In a two-and-a-half-year study, participants who responded to difficult situations with negative emotion performed less well in cognitive tests than those responding more positively.[70] The researchers believe it's the response – not the stress itself – that affects the brain.

Managing stress: we say

- Learning to manage stress is an essential life skill. Always remember that your health and happiness come first, and don't 'sweat the small stuff'.
- Cultivate a positive attitude to getting older – see Chapter 10.
- Eat to beat stress: avocados are a great source of B vitamins, which we need for a healthy nervous system; almonds contain vitamins B_2 and E, which help boost the immune system in times of stress; the vitamin C in oranges helps to lower blood pressure and the stress hormone cortisol.
- Dark chocolate (70 per cent cocoa solids or above) is believed to help reduce stress.
- Meditate: yes, it takes time, but the benefits are huge. The US Army uses it to help veterans with post-traumatic stress disorder (PTSD).
- Take a mindful walk: researchers found that students who focused on breathing and awareness of their surroundings when walking were less stressed.
- Go somewhere green. For 80 per cent of the population, greenery reduces levels of the stress hormone cortisol.[71]

Manage the menopause

Every woman on the planet – who lives long enough – will go through menopause. Yet it's a subject that's rarely discussed in public. We learn about puberty in school, childbirth in antenatal classes, and menopause, er, where?

A woman reaches menopause, technically, 12 months after her last period. But for a decade beforehand we can be in peri-menopause, when our hormones yo-yo and debilitating symptoms such as hot flushes, night sweats and mood swings can play havoc with our lives.

The process might even speed up ageing itself.[72] Data taken from more than 3,000 women analysed their biological age by looking at DNA methylation, a biomarker linked to ageing. The study found that women who had been through the men-opause were biologically older than those who hadn't, even if they were the same chronological age. 'Our study strongly sug-gests that the hormonal changes that accompany menopause accelerate biological ageing in women', the researchers wrote. They estimated that menopause speeds up cellular ageing by 6 per cent. If you take two women who are 50 years old, one of whom experienced menopause at 42, and one who has just reached it, the former would, biologically, be a year older than the latter.

To make matters worse, the same team found that the sleep issues faced by post-menopausal women are also linked to bio-logical ageing.[73] The hot flushes and restless nights common during and after menopause seem to speed up ageing. 'Not getting restorative sleep may do more than just affect our func-tioning the next day; it might also influence the rate at which our biological clock ticks,' said study researcher Judith Carroll.

What should we do? Hormone replacement therapy (HRT) has been controversial: in the early 2000s it was incorrectly linked to an increased risk of stroke, heart disease and breast cancer;[74] however, new research shows that for women with no evidence of heart disease, HRT might actually reduce risk. Nor does it cause breast, ovarian or endometrial cancer, although it might feed a tumour. (Talk to your doctor if you have a family history of breast, ovarian or endometrial cancer and are considering HRT.) Some doctors believe HRT provides more benefits than risks for most women if treatment starts before the age of 60 (or within 10 years of menopause).

Intriguingly, research shows a correlation between long-term HRT use and both increased *and* reduced risk of Alzheimer's.[75] This research hasn't been confirmed by randomised control trials, however, but it's under further investigation. JoAnn Manson, Professor of Women's Health at Harvard Medical School, told us, 'There's no clear evidence at the moment that HRT will reduce the risk of cognitive decline. There was some early evidence of less amyloid plaque in the brains of women who had taken transdermal estradiol, so now we're collaborating on a longer study.'

The menopause: we say

- If you're finding menopause tough, please, please don't suffer in silence. Talk to your nearest and dearest so that they understand. And seek help from your doctor.

- There's lots of online support from women going through the same experience. Use social media to contact other menopausal women. We like @positivepauseuk @menoandme and @megsmenopause.
- Consider simple practicalities like his-and-her single duvets rather than a double one. Sleeveless tops? A small fan in your handbag? Having a few coping strategies make us feel more in control.
- There's surprisingly little scientific research on reducing menopause symptoms with nutrition. Soya products are rich in phyto (plant) oestrogens, so they might help.
- Flax seeds also contain oestrogen-like compounds: we add them, ground, to porridge and smoothies.
- Exercise and keeping body weight under control might help with symptoms. It's easy to reach for a sugary snack when you're feeling tired, but sugar adds to menopausal fatigue – as well as weight gain.
- Avoid refined carbs: when you're feeling low and moody, a blood-sugar roller coaster is the last thing you need. The same goes for caffeine. Menopause leads to disturbed sleep, so avoid caffeine after 2pm.
- Spicy food causes our body temperature to rise – not what you want if you're already suffering with hot flushes. Try chilled fruit and salads instead.
- Lower oestrogen levels impact our bones, so make sure you're getting enough calcium and vitamin D. They also affect heart health, so eating plenty of fibre coupled with a reduced intake of saturated fats is important.

- Too much alcohol is best avoided; however, research shows that the polyphenols found in hops and beer can help to alleviate symptoms.[76] Seek out a lower alcohol beer, and enjoy it cold!
- The advice from the Royal College of GPs remains, 'best practice for most women is to prescribe the lowest possible dose of hormones for the shortest possible time in order to achieve satisfactory relief of symptoms'.

CHAPTER 2

Create Your Own Health Portrait

Now that you understand how and why the human body ages, you might want to assess your own unique risk factors. These are the factors unique to you, either genetic or as a result of earlier lifestyle choices, like smoking or heavy drinking. Every individual is different, which means that we each have our own risk profile, our health strengths and weaknesses. It's not essential, but creating a health portrait enables us to more accurately focus our Age-Well efforts. It also provides a benchmark from which to monitor progress. This section explains how you can better understand your personal risk profile and your current state of health, by creating a health portrait.

Gather together the necessary information

In a nutshell, you should know: what your recent ancestors suffered or died from and at roughly what age; diseases in your immediate family; risk factors thrown up by your DNA; your current blood pressure level; waist-to-hip ratio; your cholesterol level; and your blood sugar/glucose levels. We also suggest keeping an eye on your resting heart rate. Your GP or the nurse at your GP's surgery can help with these tests. DNA testing kits will provide basic gene analysis. Ask the older members of your family for help with ancestral information.

We started our Age-Well Project by compiling ancestral health trees, listing the ageing diseases, causes of mortality and ages at death of as many direct ancestors and family members as possible. We added any other relevant facts (a history of smoking or drinking, career details, war injuries, and so on) that might help us to explain how well – or not – they aged. We keep these pinned to our walls to help us stay on track.

We then did DNA tests from the biotechnology company, 23andme. Annabel's DNA analysis highlighted some of the conditions her parents and grandparents had suffered from. Susan's analysis showed a variant of the ApoE4 gene, which increases her risk of Alzheimer's disease. These results, coupled with a portrait of our ancestral health patterns, gave us a clearer sense of our genetic risk factors.

We then had our blood pressure, blood glucose, cholesterol and vitamin D levels tested, as well as our bone density (sometimes called a DEXA), and a full blood count. Finally, we updated our waist-to-hip ratios and our BMI. These provided a picture of our current health which, married with our ancestral findings and DNA results, helped us to devise more personalised Age-Well plans.

If we – two busy working mums – can do this, so can you. This is where we started and what we did, and we recommend you do it too:

- Put together a health tree of your ancestors, adding their age at death, cause of death and any known illnesses in old age.
- Have your genotype tested. Download the full raw data set, then upload it to a secondary service for more in-depth analysis (we used Promethease which cost $12 at time of writing, but there are many others). Be prepared to spend several hours getting to grips with your personal data – this is complicated information and the data can run to tens of pages.
- Know your current blood pressure, your body mass index (BMI) and waist-to-hip ratio (WHR), your resting heart rate, your cholesterol levels, and your blood glucose levels. We have these basic tests done – for free, or rather included in our membership – every few months at our gym (www.nuffield.com). They're not essential, but they provide a good starting point and a benchmark against which to monitor progress. Besides, dangerously high and/or low levels of any of these will need addressing.
- If your cholesterol is high, ask for a more in-depth lipid panel to test separate LDL and HDL levels.
- If you've a family history of broken bones and osteoporosis, ask your GP to refer you for a bone density scan and a vitamin D test.
- If you've a family history of inflammatory disease (which includes cancer, Alzheimer's and any autoimmune

disease), ask for a C-reactive protein (CRP) test. This measures the amount of inflammation in your body.

- If you're concerned about vitamin deficiencies, ask for a full vitamin screen/profile. If you're concerned about iron deficiency (or having too much iron, which can be dangerous as we age), ask for a complete blood count.
- Keep up to date with smears, mammograms and colonoscopies.
- Please be aware that some GPs might be reluctant to order these if they see no reason for them (even as part of a preventative Age-Well programme).

There are many other tests that you can take to see how well you're ageing, from telomere measurements to full hormone analyses, but for the purpose of building your own Age-Well plan, the above should suffice unless you have specific conditions. As usual, always discuss with your GP in the first instance.

Have your genes tested

Geneticists now believe that 50–90 per cent of the signs and diseases of ageing are caused by lifestyle. This gives us huge scope to improve our lot: the genetic code adapted by our ancestors over millions of years and passed to us at birth. Of course, our DNA is our personal blueprint for ageing. But that's all it is: a blueprint. We now know that the expression of our genes can be modified by exercise, diet, sleep, stress and other lifestyle factors, a process studied and known as epigenetics. We all have the power to change how our genes are expressed – just as we might modify a blueprint for a new house by changing the door handles or increasing the size of the windows.

Our Age-Well Project is designed for anyone wanting to defy the usual diseases of ageing, regardless of their DNA; however, we found having our genes tested both helpful and motivating.* A recent study mirrors this, suggesting that giving individuals access to their genetic data leads to more vigilant and sustained efforts at lifestyle changes. As the author said, 'we believe giving information on their genetic profile to individuals is particularly motivating.'[1]

Knowing our genetic risks encouraged us to modify our personal Age-Well programmes. Annabel's high genetic risk of deep-vein thrombosis made her re-think long-haul flights: she now wears compression stockings and walks the aisle every 30 minutes. She thinks twice about driving long distances, preferring to take the train. Her gene test also nudged her into investing in a treadmill desk, where much of this book was written.

Meanwhile, Susan is focusing her Age-Well Project on brain health after discovering she carries the ApoE4 variant, putting her at an increased risk of Alzheimer's. She's also taking more

---

* Note: 23andme, ancestry.com and other consumer gene-testing providers offer a genotyping service, which means they report on only a fraction of your DNA (think of this DNA as the major pit stops on a motorway). There are two other options, although both are considerably more expensive and may need to be ordered via a healthcare provider. Whole Genome Sequencing (WGS) is undoubtedly the future and involves sequencing your full DNA (on our motorway analogy, this means reporting on every pit stop, every exit/entrance and every piece of hard shoulder along the way). It's costly, not really designed for consumers (yet) and might not provide much more than its cheaper genotyping counterpart, as we write. Finally, there's Whole Exome Sequencing (WES) which sequences only the parts of DNA coding for proteins, so that's more than genotyping and less than WGS (on our motorway analogy, that would mean major pit stops, all the exits/entrances – including those no one's ever heard of – but not the hard shoulder). Our advice is to use one of the popular genotyping services for now.

rigorous care of her eyes after discovering her genetic disposition for age-related macular degeneration: upping her daily intake of yellow/orange vegetables, wearing sunglasses more regularly and quitting her 4am Instagram scrolling, among other things.

The cost of basic gene-testing is around £140 at the time of writing, but some companies offer big discounts on National DNA Day, April 25, the anniversary of the day the human genome project was completed. We fully expect the cost of gene testing to continue to fall.

Once your data's been returned, you'll need to run it through a secondary service. We used Promethease, which we found to be particularly comprehensive and easy to navigate. We suggest doing additional research only on those genes where mutation has considerably raised your risk. But remember, this is only a heightened risk factor compared to the population average, not a conclusion. Never forget that you can alter the expression of your genes.

If your results suggest a genetic predisposition for a chronic condition or disease, use this as an incentive to become better informed. There are lots of support groups and online forums (like apoe4.info if you have the so-called 'Alzheimer's gene'), often packed with useful information.

Lastly, rejoice in your good genes. But don't take them for granted. You might not have the fatso gene, but that doesn't mean you can gorge yourself on doughnuts every day. Nor does not having the ApoE4 gene make you immune to Alzheimer's.

The field of genes and epigenetics is huge, complex and fast moving. Entire books have been written on the subject, and if you want to know more, we recommend reading works by those who've studied extensively in this field. Please refer to our reading list at the end of this book.

Your genes: we say

- Consider having your genes tested (unless it's going to make you anxious).
- Cross-check your results with your ancestral health tree, looking for patterns.
- Modify your own Age-Well Project accordingly.
- Remember, you can alter the expression of your genes through lifestyle choices.

CORNERSTONE ONE

Diet

Nothing impacts our health more than our diet, so this is where our Age-Well Project began. Knowing we can make a difference to our longevity with what we eat has proved empowering and uplifting. The food we put into our bodies fuels every cell, and as we grow older, the quality of this fuel becomes ever more important. We need fewer calories, so each one has to count.

The risks of developing any of the chronic diseases of ageing are significantly reduced by healthy eating. The highest quality diet (which includes full-fat dairy and, yes, red meat) is linked to a 25 per cent lower risk of death when compared to the lowest-quality diet, packed with refined carbohydrate.[1]

Poor diet is linked to heart disease, diabetes and increased inflammation. Obesity is the second biggest cancer risk after smoking. Older adults who eat at least one portion of green leafy vegetables each day have the slowest rate of cognitive decline.[2] To age well, we must eat well.

Diet

CHAPTER 3

How to Eat

Our research showed that we needed to change not only what we ate, but *how*, *when* and *where* we ate. Food is a powerful tool: we've learnt to use it wisely.

In the next few chapters we discuss several significant studies of diet and ageing. To make this information easier to navigate and absorb, 'We say' boxes summarise the changes we've made over the last five years. Pick one change at a time (choosing the easiest and most appealing first) to make the process less daunting. For an overview, see also our brief explanation of the diet section in the Introduction.

From processed food to a Mediterranean-style diet

In five years, our Age-Well Project has transformed every facet of how we feed ourselves and our families. The once ubiquitous evening meal of white pasta, pesto (from a jar) and frozen peas has long been replaced by several vegetable dishes (three or four at every meal, but none taking more than a few minutes to prepare) generously embellished with herbs and spices and gleaming with extra virgin olive oil. We usually include some animal protein – often fish or eggs – and invariably a pulse or an interesting whole grain. Packets of breakfast cereal rarely make it into the larder. Commercially made biscuits are a hazy memory. Crisps have been replaced with our own herby roasted nuts or home-popped corn. We, and our families, are eating better than ever before – if we say so ourselves.

If we fancy steak and chips, a plate of prosciutto or a muffin, we have it – but not very often and rarely from a plastic packet. We can honestly say we've never felt deprived (or guilty, for that matter). For us, eating a plant-based diet is a joy rather than a hardship.

If we hadn't enjoyed cooking (and poring over cookery books), changing how we ate would have been considerably harder. On this point, we must be crystal clear: if you learn to cook – and to love the process of cooking – changing how you eat will be a pleasure rather than a chore. It will also be the most important thing you can do to nurture your longevity. We can't put it any better than food writer Bee Wilson, in *This is Not a Diet Book: A User's Guide to Eating Well*: 'Cooking is the best way to take control of your own nourishment.'

Many other factors helped our transition to a Mediterranean-style of eating. We became liberal and adventurous users of herbs and spices. By making our food fully flavoured, we were able to match the intensity of commercially processed food with its 'proven' holy trinity of fat, sugar and salt (perfected by food scientists in all things salted caramel). This helped to give our meals child-appeal as well as placating our husbands as we weaned them from their preference for meat-heavy meals. We never shied away from using butter, salt and cream (in moderation). Not only do we think these have been unduly demonised but they often make dishes taste better (strawberries and cream is a pudding that can hardly be improved upon, while melted butter on asparagus or a swirl of cream in soup can only be a good thing).

Time – for shopping, preparation and eating

As busy working mothers, our greatest challenge was finding time: the time to shop, prep, cook and clear up. We overcame this by keeping well-stocked freezers (peas, edamame beans, spinach, home-made stock, lemons) and larders (pre-cooked pulses of every sort, tinned tomatoes, spice mixes, seeds and nuts) and building a list of dishes that involve minimal ingredients and can be cooked in minutes (see the selection of recipes at the end of the book and visit our blog for more). We frequently cook double portions and freeze half so that we always have a 'ready meal' to hand, and we often prep or cook supper as we're making breakfast for our children, always lavishing as much attention on the vegetables as on any main part of the dish. Incidentally, we use smaller plates now (and smaller wine glasses) to prevent over-eating (and – ahem – over-drinking).

In the old days, we habitually ate at any time between 8pm and 10pm, but now we try to eat three hours before bedtime (circumstances permitting). We've also pushed back our breakfasts to be as late as possible, enabling a longer overnight fast; research increasingly links a longer period of time between meals with healthy longevity, perhaps because it gives our bodies more time for rest and repair.[1] Fruit juice has become an occasional treat rather than the routine purchase it once was. Instead, we eat whole fruit, giving us the benefits of fibre (and the full range of nutrients) without excess sugar.

Not eating in a pre-bed or early morning rush has also enabled us to eat more slowly, something Director of Research at Norwich Medical School, Professor Anne-Marie Minihane, believes is an essential, but overlooked, factor in the Mediterranean diet. She told us, 'The original Med diet isn't only about food. It's the whole lifestyle. Here we tend to eat very fast and I urge people to slow down. Our satiety hormones don't kick in for 20 minutes, by which time most people have over-eaten. In the Mediterranean they eat more socially, which is always slower.'[2]

We've stopped our snacking and grazing habits too. According to Dr Dawn Harper, people who graze underestimate their daily calorific intake by 500–1,000 calories a day.[3] But, equally detrimental, constant snacking means that the digestive system is *permanently* working and we're *permanently* producing insulin, potentially leading to insulin resistance. According to neurologist Dr David Perlmutter, anything that promotes insulin resistance raises our risk of Alzheimer's. Meanwhile, nephrologist Dr Jason Fung urges us to eat only at mealtimes, as our ancestors did.[4]

Our shopping habits changed to reflect these dietary shifts. We found the easiest way to stick to our new eating style was not to have snacks or processed food in the house – at all. We also made changes to how we cooked. In particular we reduced the quantities of sugar in our baking, often by 50 per cent. All too often no one noticed.

Puddings – which used to appear religiously after every meal – became weekend and holiday treats. There was initial resistance, inevitably, but children are generally much more adaptable than we like to think.

Finally, we keep an eye on how often we eat out (and that includes a sandwich on the run). Like everyone, we love a restaurant, particularly for a special occasion. But is it any coincidence that the rise of obesity, type-2 diabetes and other chronic disease mirrors the rise of food outlets? As children, we ate out on birthdays (if we were lucky). Today over a third of Brits eat out once or twice a week, with many younger people ordering takeaway pizza several times a month.[5] Mass-catered food isn't like the food we cook at home. The chances are it includes more refined sugar, fat and salt.

Cooking and eating habits: we say

- Learn to cook. Not elaborate fussy dishes, but everyday meals that can be whipped up in less than half an hour. Take a course if you need to, but today's cookery books are clear, easy-to-follow and glossily inspiring, while YouTube is awash with cooking tutorials. Alternatively, take a look at our website agewellproject.com.
- Have the right equipment. A good knife and a food processor that blends, slices and grates (indispensable for making fast slaws and soups) will pay for itself within months.
- A cheap salad spinner enables us to avoid salad bags and use the full, fresher lettuce.
- Don't have food/drink in the house that you no longer want to eat or drink – you may not be able to resist it: out of sight is out of mind.
- Remove things over time, rather than throwing out all

the processed food in one go. We got rid of crisps and
processed biscuits first, followed by refined breakfast
cereals and sweetened yoghurts.

- Experiment with reducing sugar when you bake.
- Eat with others – using smaller plates and smaller glasses.
- Make your meals look beautiful: edible flowers, zest,
  chopped herbs, sprinkled nuts, colour, and so on.
- Unless you have blood sugar levels that rise and fall
  quickly, avoid snacking and grazing.
- Eat three hours before bed and leave a good 12 hours
  before your next meal.
- Give the ubiquitous 'meal deal' a miss and take a
  lunchbox to work.
- An omelette and a salad takes as long to prepare as a
  ready-meal – and is infinitely more delicious and conducive
  to ageing well!

Should we care about calories?

For many of us, calorie counting has become a way of life. It's
very rare for us to pick up a pack or jar in the supermarket and
not check, almost instinctively, its calories. The calorific value of
a food is only a way of measuring the amount of energy it produces when burnt, but the word has become laden with meaning
and guilt. As part of this Project, we've learnt to let go of that
guilt and focus on the nutrient value of food instead.

When it comes to ageing well, there are two conflicting
approaches to calories: on one hand there's compelling evidence

that counting calories is not the answer to weight loss; on the other hand research suggests calorie restriction might be an elixir of youth.

We grew up with the idea of 'calories in, calories out'. Eat more calories than you burn, and you'll gain weight. Burn more calories than you eat, and you'll lose weight; however, our Age-Well Project has taught us what an over-simplification this is. Our bodies respond differently to different foods. Give them doughnuts and out races insulin to manage the sugar rush. Consequently, the calories are stored as fat. Give them healthy fats, vegetables and fibre and they respond very differently. As Dr Mark Hyman says in *Eat Fat, Get Thin*: 'Food, it turns out, is not just calories, but *information* that radically influences our genes, hormones, immune system, brain chemistry, and even gut flora with every single bite.'

Maintaining a healthy weight helps us to age well. It's not about being thin but, as you'll have read in Chapter 1, having a good waist-to-hip ratio. Obesity is one of the main drivers of diabetes and the second highest risk factor for cancer (after smoking). Many doctors and nutritionists believe that there's no point in counting calories, and that reducing refined carbohydrate intake is the best way to lose weight.

Some scientists have become increasingly vocal on the role of calorie restriction (CR) in healthy ageing. Long-term studies show that a 20–40 per cent reduction in calories promotes longevity. Calorie restriction, like intermittent fasting, appears to trigger autophagy, the process by which our bodies burn up damaged cells.

The subjects of these long-term studies are animals, not humans. A 25-year study of monkeys on a reduced-calorie diet (30 per cent fewer calories than they previously consumed) found a major increase in longevity and a reduction in age-related illness.[6] Similar studies in yeast, dogs, flies and rodents found an increase of roughly 40 per cent in longevity. Researchers have estimated that for humans, the increase could be five to ten years.

Research has also shown that calorie restriction might impact brain health. In another animal study, mice were fed food pellets with 30 per cent fewer calories. The impact on their hippocampus (a part of the brain considered vital for learning and memory) was measured for a year.[7] The calorie restriction suppressed the gene expression that normally results in brain ageing. The lead researcher suggested it adds 'evidence for the role of diet in delaying the effects of ageing and age-related disease'.

These are interesting studies, and while we'd love another five to ten years of healthy life, we don't want to go hungry. Equally, living on 30 per cent fewer calories impacts our health in other ways, particularly our bone mass. Not to mention feeling 'hangry' (hungry + angry), which affects feelings of positivity and purpose, also critical as we age. This is why we focus on eating *quality* food, rather than cutting calories.

Calories and hunger: we say

- Research is at an early stage, but there's evidence that a low-protein, high-carbohydrate diet can mimic the effects of calorie restriction in mice[8] by increasing lifespan and improving blood sugar.
- Food shouldn't be a source of guilt. Never count calories. Instead eat unprocessed, high-fibre foods.

- If you're struggling with your weight, talk to your GP.
- Read the section on intermittent fasting (on page 76), which has many of the benefits of calorie restriction without the hunger. We prefer to leave a longer gap between dinner and breakfast than get hangry.

Why we put plants front and centre (but still eat animal products)

If we had just one piece of dietary advice for your personal Age-Well Project, it would be this: eat more plants. Many of the largest studies into diet and longevity confirm the importance of plant-based foods, showing that *upping* our intake of vegetables, fruits, nuts, pulses and grains, while *reducing* our intake of meat and saturated fat drastically improves health.

Walter Willett, Professor of Epidemiology and Nutrition at the Harvard School of Public Health, stated at a conference in 2018, 'We've just been doing some calculations looking at the question of how much could we reduce mortality by shifting towards a healthy, more plant-based diet, not necessarily totally vegan, and our estimates are about one third of deaths could be prevented.'

A 2018 study revealed an interesting experiment in which researchers analysed dietary data from over 11,700 participants. They constructed their own 'plant-based diet index', which assigned positive scores for plant foods and negative scores for animal foods. They then allocated marks for 'healthful' plant-based foods. When the researchers looked at causes of death among the participants, they found a 5 per cent reduction in risk of death from all causes among the healthful plant-based eaters.[9]

Plant-based eating appears to be particularly beneficial in reducing cardiovascular disease risk. When researchers reviewed data from over 70,000 American women they found that those who followed a diet based on whole grains, nuts and vegetables had a substantially lower risk of heart disease than those following a diet heavy on crisps, sweets and fizzy drinks.[10]

We've put vegetables front and centre in our Age-Well diets, not on the side of our plates. This has meant eating more plant protein from beans, legumes, pulses, nuts and seeds. A 2016 study, reviewing nutritional data from over 130,000 people found that those who consumed more plant-based protein lived longer than those who ate large amounts of meat and eggs. A 3 per cent increase in calories from plant protein reduced the risk of death from all causes by 10 per cent. It's a good reason to replace some animal protein with more plant protein.

We typically make at least three-quarters of our food intake plant-based. We don't avoid animal products, but we try to make them organic when we can – quality not quantity.[11]

Plants and pulses: we say

- Aim for your plate to be two-thirds plant based.
- If you eat meat and dairy, think about how you can work more plant protein into your diet.

- We eat generous amounts of pulses (peas, beans and lentils) and nuts. See the recipe section at the end of the book and check our blog for inspiration.
- Meat is an occasional treat for us, as it is for many of the world's longest-lived people. Blue Zoners eat meat and/or fish, but not every day.

Eat organic

Fewer chemicals mean better health. We eat organically whenever we can (for various reasons not limited to our health) but we know this isn't possible for everyone. If you have access to – and can afford – organic food or a little space to grow your own, research suggests that this might be a simple way to reduce the burden of chemicals on your ageing body and brain while increasing the nutrients in your food.

For those who find it harder to rid their bodies of toxins (cancer patients and carriers of certain genes that make detoxification more difficult), eating organically is worth considering. We need more research, as scientists still don't understand what happens when multiple chemicals accumulate and interact (the cocktail effect) over an extended period of time. As Professor Minihane told us: 'We just don't know what the long-term effects of ingesting pesticides will be.'

We do know, however, that industrial-style farming has left vast tracts of farmland depleted of nutrients – and that means less nutrient-dense fruit, vegetables, meat and dairy. In the UK, between 1940 and 1990 copper levels in vegetables fell by 76 per cent and calcium by 46 per cent. The amount of protein, phosphorous, iron, riboflavin (B_2) and vitamin C also fell.

It's no surprise, then, that a meta-analysis of 343 studies into the compositional differences between organic and non-organic crops found that switching to organic fruit, vegetables and cereals (and food produced thereof) provided additional antioxidants equivalent to eating one to two extra portions of fruit and vegetables a day.[12] More specifically, the researchers found organic produce to be 51 per cent higher in anthocyanins, 50 per cent higher in flavonols, 69 per cent higher in flavanones and 26 per cent higher in flavones (each of which is an antioxidant vital for ageing well).

The same study also found that organic crops had significantly lower levels of toxic metals, with contamination from cadmium – previously linked to kidney and bone disease – being 50 per cent lower. Indeed, pesticide residues were four times less likely to be found in organic crops; however, arsenic and lead levels were almost the same in both organic and conventional crops.

Organically fed cows produce milk and meat that's typically 50 per cent higher in omega-3s than conventionally fed cows.[13] Organic milk and dairy also contain slightly higher concentrations of iron, vitamin E and some carotenoids.

The good news is that one can glean most of the benefits of an organic diet without going the whole hog. Some fruit and vegetables are consistently more contaminated, either because their skins enable greater chemical saturation or because they're subject to heavier use of pesticides and fertilisers. By avoiding the worst offenders, we can substantially reduce our ingestion of pesticides.

In the United States these crops, known as the Dirty Dozen and the Clean Fifteen, are reviewed every year and made public at www.ewg.org. In Europe, pesticide regulation and usage can differ, so our cleanest and dirtiest crops will also differ (and in fact our more stringent laws provide us with greater protection than our American counterparts). The latest pesticide review[14] has identified the UK's dirtiest and cleanest fruit and vegetables (you can read the full list, which also includes grains and meat at http://www.pan-uk.org/our-food/). We've extrapolated a UK Dirty Dozen and EU Clean Fifteen, as follows (and in order, so that those found to carry the greatest concentration of pesticide residues are listed first):

UK Dirty Dozen

- citrus (oranges, lemons and so on)
- strawberries
- pears
- grapes
- herbs
- apples
- cherries
- peaches and nectarines
- pineapples
- apricots

- bananas
- pre-prepared salad

EU Clean Fifteen

- beetroot
- cauliflower
- corn-on-the-cob
- figs
- mushrooms
- onions
- rhubarb
- swede
- turnip
- peas in pods (mange-tout)
- spring onions
- asparagus
- radishes
- avocados
- peas

Choosing fruit and veg: we say

- We keep lists of the 'dirtiest' and 'cleanest' produce pinned up in our kitchens. Equally, we try not to become too stressed over our consumption of non-organic food, because we know that stress might be equally damaging.
- Try growing some of the easier-to-grow fruit and vegetables – apples, courgettes, chard, cucumbers, rhubarb and beans are favourites in our garden.
- Herbs are highly sprayed. Try growing your own in pots on the windowsill.
- Grapes are heavily sprayed, so we've switched to drinking organic or biodynamic wine. It may cost a little more, but we drink less of it – so it all balances out in the end.
- We rarely buy non-organic meat now, but, as we've cut our meat consumption, the higher cost of organic meat hasn't affected our weekly food budget.
- Can't find the organic produce you want? Ask your supermarket to consider stocking it, or use an organic veg box delivery service.

Intermittent fasting

The word 'fasting' fills people with horror – who wants to be hungry? However, a mounting body of research links fasting to healthy longevity. Let's be clear: this isn't long-term fasting, which makes daily life impossible. This is short-term, daily fasting, known as intermittent fasting, which we've found easy to work into our daily lives. And it's big news: reports show its beneficial effects on everything from type-2 diabetes to Alzheimer's.

Intermittent fasting – or IF – can take many forms:

- You may have heard of the 5:2 diet (eat normally for five days a week, and eat 500–600 calories for two days). The weight-loss elements of the diet were originally a happy side effect of author Michael Mosley's research into longevity.
- There are other variants: the 16:8 diet promotes eating a whole day's calories in an eight-hour window, then fasting for the remaining 16 hours.
- A research project found that participants lost weight by eating 25 per cent of their daily calorie allowance on one day, and 175 per cent the next.[15]
- Dr Valter Longo, whose work on longevity and fasting inspired the 5:2 diet, has his own version: a five-day fast-mimicking diet which allows 800 calories a day of nuts, oil and vegetables. It's just enough food to keep you going, but not enough to trigger insulin production, thereby tricking the body into fasting mode.
- Other forms are even simpler: don't eat for at least 12 hours a day. This is the preferred method of Dr Dale Bredesen in his protocol for people suffering from mild cognitive impairment. He also advises not eating three hours before bedtime.

Although each method is slightly different, they all aim for the same result: a state of autophagy in the body. The term 'autophagy' literally means 'eating of self'. At its simplest, this is the body spring-cleaning itself: clearing up damaged cells and proteins in the body and brain.[16] This process accelerates when the body is in a fasted state. It takes the body about 12 hours to use up glucose stored in the liver. At this point autophagy kicks in, and the clean-up starts. Old damaged cells provide energy to other cells, helping them regenerate.

Research has linked autophagy to a variety of healthy ageing benefits:

Reduced risk of type-2 diabetes During intermittent fasting, blood sugar levels decrease – as do insulin levels. This means that insulin stands by ready to spring into action next time we eat, rather than constantly coursing through our body and potentially making us insulin resistant – a pre-cursor to diabetes (as previously explained on page 37).[17]

Protection against Alzheimer's disease A build-up of beta-amyloid plaque in the brain has long been linked to Alzheimer's. Researchers have found that IF helped the brain clean up amyloid.[18]

The possible slowing of tumour growth in cancer This is subject to on-going research, but it seems that a group of proteins, sirtuins, is activated by fasting and might slow tumour growth.[19]

Fasting and hunger: we say

- Leave at least 12 hours between dinner and breakfast – up to 16 if it suits you.

- Make a quick breakfast pot before bed, so that you can grab it and go in the morning. Mix oats, chia seeds, cinnamon, milk and berries, and leave them to soak overnight. Vary it by adding different toppings in the morning: banana slices, cacao powder, defrosted cherries, probiotic yoghurt or nut butter.
- Avoid eating late in the evening.
- Don't eat between meals.
- Don't be frightened of hunger. This isn't the same as dieting – we know we're going to get food soon. But can you go another hour without eating? You probably can.

The best nutrition for bone density

Our bones are extraordinary: they are constantly remodelling and rebuilding themselves throughout our lives. In our twenties, damage from wear and tear is replaced, so our bones remain strong. But as we age, they're not rebuilt at the same rate and they start to weaken, a condition known as osteopenia. Their structure becomes increasingly honeycombed: holey and sponge-like. If this becomes extreme, osteoporosis (literally: porous bones) can result. Weakened bones are more likely to fracture, particularly at the hip, spine and ankle but, luckily, there's plenty we can do to reduce the risk.

Some people are more likely to get osteoporosis than others: smoking, alcohol consumption, low body weight and genetics all play a part. Calcium intake is also crucial. Ninety-nine per cent of our calcium is in our bones, but popping a pill is not necessarily the answer. Research shows that our bones absorb dietary calcium better than calcium from supplements.[20]

How, then, do we get dietary calcium? It's wrong to assume that dairy products are the only source. Bony fish such as sardines provide good levels of calcium. And it's perfectly possible to get all the calcium we need from plant sources. Calcium finds its way into plants from the earth, ending up in dairy products because cows eat plants. The calcium in plants is easier for our bodies to absorb than the calcium in milk. Brassicas such as pak choi, kale and broccoli are rich in calcium. Eat lots of calcium-rich foods and you'll have the bones of an elephant, right? Well, not quite.

Australian research found that women over 55 who ate more vegetables, particularly brassicas and alliums (onions, garlic, leeks, and so on), had a lower fracture risk.[21] The research team suggested that this might be because, in addition to calcium, these vegetables contain many of the other nutrients needed to build strong bones; for example, brassicas are also a good source of vitamin K, which has been linked to a lower incidence of hip fracture. A compound called sulforaphane, found abundantly in both cruciferous and allium vegetables, has been shown to help build strong bones.

Nutrients for strong bones are:

- calcium
- vitamin D
- magnesium
- vitamin C
- vitamin E
- vitamin K

- boron
- vitamin B$_{12}$ and folate
- isoflavones

Bone health: we say

Eat for your bones:

- Salmon and eggs provide vitamin D.
- Whole grains, quinoa and spinach for magnesium.
- Citrus fruit for vitamin C.
- Avocados for vitamin E.
- Dark leafy greens for vitamin K.
- Chickpeas, beans and almonds for boron.
- Soya for isoflavones.
- We love tinned sardines (with the bones) for calcium. We eat them on toast for a quick and thrifty lunch.

Don't be afraid of the sun – try to get plenty of daylight to boost your vitamin D levels.

Fibre

We all grew up knowing we should eat fibre. 'Fibre keeps you regular' was the mantra of the 1970s. True, but it also does plenty more.

Government guidelines in the UK suggest adults need 30g of fibre a day. That's a lot. And we aren't getting enough: the average UK consumption is just 18g per person. As part of our Age-Well Project we've tracked our fibre intake and worked hard to ensure we're getting enough. We've found eating 30g a day difficult; however, as we're both quite petite, 25g is perfectly acceptable and achievable.

Fibre is an indigestible, plant-based carbohydrate. The richest sources are whole grains, pulses (peas, beans and lentils), vegetables, fruit and nuts. You may have heard the terms 'soluble' and 'insoluble' fibre in the past. Soluble fibre is soft and bulks up with water to form a gel that passes through the body; insoluble fibre is the roughage that passes through the digestive tract, sweeping out waste as it goes. These terms aren't used as much by doctors now, because fibre-rich foods usually contain both types. In fact, there may be many more types of fibre all doing roughly the same thing.

Fibre has many jobs in our bodies:

Reducing cholesterol levels, which helps heart health. A soluble fibre, beta glucan, binds with bile acids and helps the body to excrete them. When the body needs to make more bile acids, it uses cholesterol from the blood, and levels go down.

Protecting against diabetes Carbohydrate from high-fibre foods is absorbed more slowly into the bloodstream, keeping blood sugar and insulin levels stable.

Controlling weight Fibre keeps us feeling fuller for longer.

Lowering colorectal cancer risk It seems that by moving the food through the gut quickly, fibre reduces the amount of time waste is in contact with the bowel. The World Cancer Research Fund estimates that 45 per cent of bowel cancer could be prevented through diet, physical activity and weight control.

Reducing inflammation (see page 30).

An Australian study looked at the carbohydrates consumed by 1,600 healthy people aged 49 and above and followed them for ten years. The researchers wanted to see if the cohort would be 'successful agers', defined as 'being free of disability and chronic disease (coronary artery disease, stroke, diabetes, and cancer); having good mental health and functional independence; and having good physical, respiratory, and cognitive function'. After ten years, the most successful agers were those who consumed the most fibre. The fibre source was usually fruit, wholegrain bread and cereals such as oats. The researchers suggest two possible reasons for this:

1   A link between inflammation, insulin production and ageing. Inflammation occurs when the body produces free radicals in response to the flood of insulin triggered by a meal high in sugar and refined carbohydrate. Fibre slows this process, keeping our insulin levels on an even keel and keeping inflammation at bay.
2   Some types of fibre, known as resistant starch, ferment in the gut. Our gut microbiota create a fermentation process, which produces short-chain fatty acids. These fatty acids also work to reduce inflammation in the body.[22]

Fibre: we say

- Keep a fibre diary to ensure you're getting sufficient. Half a tin of baked beans contains 7.5g of fibre, a medium avocado contains 4.5g of fibre; a large banana 3.6g; a 75g serving of barley 3g; 3 Weetabix 5.4g; 100g cooked red kidney beans 6.2g.
- Try to get as close to 30g a day as you can.
- Read food labels to calculate the quantity of fibre in your diet.
- Review your daily intake of fibre and make sure you're eating quality carbohydrates. Whole grains such as brown rice, quinoa and granary bread, contain more fibre than white bread, pasta and rice.
- Eat oats and barley, both are rich in beta glucans.
- If you increase your fibre intake too quickly, you might feel bloated and uncomfortable. Take it slowly.
- Make sure you drink plenty of water to keep all that fibre moving through your system.

Good fats, bad fats: which type and how much?

Fat is one of the most divisive subjects we've researched. UK government dietary guidelines say that no more than 35 per cent of our daily energy intake should come from fat, of which no more than 11 per cent should come from saturated fat. And yet best-selling books like *The Big Fat Surprise* (Nina Teicholz), *Grain Brain* (David Perlmutter) and *Eat Fat, Get Thin* (Mark

Hyman) recommend a high-fat, low-carb diet for better health and longevity. These books, and the research behind them, reveal the failure of low-fat diets peddled for the last 50 years. As Nina Teicholz says in *The Big Fat Surprise*, the 'low-fat diet, it turns out, has been terrible for health in every way, as evidenced by skyrocketing rates of obesity and diabetes and the failure to conquer heart disease'.

Manufacturers of low-fat foods often replaced fat with highly refined carbohydrates, and herein lies the problem. Low-fat yoghurts, for example, often contain more sugar than their full-fat counterparts. A wide-ranging meta-analysis involving data from 18 countries concluded that higher carbohydrate intake was linked to a higher risk of death. The same study found no link between total fat intake and heart disease, effectively turning years of low-fat hype on its head. Unsurprisingly, the researchers recommended that 'global dietary guidelines should be reconsidered'.[23]

When Harvard researchers recently tried to 'transcend the diet wars' and find common ground between the various factions – low-fat, low-carb, keto, Paleo – they focused on *quality* of fats rather than quantity. They dismissed the notion that fats should account for an exact proportion of our calorie intake, saying, 'We have strong evidence that the percent of calories from fat in the diet is much less important than the type of fat.'[24] This was music to our ears: focus on the *quality* of fats rather than worrying about the quantity. This means sticking to less processed fats like olive oil, avocados and nuts, while avoiding heavily processed, 'industrial' fats like seed oils.

The very worst of the 'industrial' fats are trans fats, which raise the level of 'bad' cholesterol in our blood. When vegetable oils are processed by hydrogenation (for use in margarine and commercially produced biscuits, for example), they become trans fats. Research in New York State found that people living in districts that restricted trans fats were less likely to be hospitalised for heart attack and stroke.[25] Food manufacturers and supermarkets have since phased out the use of almost all trans fats, and there are calls for a global ban. But trans fats are also produced when ordinary oils are heated to very high temperatures, as in the frying process used in fast-food production (see the section later in this chapter for more on cooking methods).

When we talked to Professor Meir Stampfer of Harvard, he said: 'If you ask "is butter bad for me?" the answer has to be, "Compared to what?" Compared to olive oil, the answer's yes, but compared to trans fats, the answer's no. We don't know all the factors that make food good or bad for us yet.' In the meantime, he uses olive oil.

Fats: we say

- We love unsaturated plant-based 'good' fats such as avocado, nuts and olive oil, because they come with a host of health benefits.
- Avocados are a rich source of fibre as well as the carotenoids lutein and zeaxanthin, which are good for eye health and for reducing osteoarthritis risk.
- Nuts are also full of fibre and minerals such as selenium and calcium.
- Olive oil is liquid gold packed with antioxidant polyphenols to protect the heart.
- Research indicates dairy products are heart protective, particularly when they are cultured or fermented, for

example probiotic yoghurt or kefir. Full-fat yoghurt tastes so much better than the low-fat version. Probiotic yoghurt benefits gut health, too.

- Don't skimp on the salad dressing: oils like olive, avocado and walnut help the body absorb nutrients from the leaves. Avoid sunflower oil though (see page 101).
- Drizzle a little olive oil over steamed green vegetables for the same reason.
- Experiment with oils for dressing and drizzling: avocado, walnut and hazelnut oils all add flavour.
- Different oils have different uses: use regular olive oil for light frying and save the extra-virgin for drizzling and dressings.
- Vitamins A, D, E and K are fat-soluble, so we can only absorb them if we're consuming fats too.
- Avoid fried fast food. And when frying at home, keep temperatures as low as possible.
- Do you enjoy butter? Go ahead, but in moderation.

Watch the salt, but don't panic

Salt: another contentious area where medics and researchers rarely agree. Is salt good for us, or bad for us? Reports say both. Higher levels of salt have been linked, bafflingly, to both higher *and* lower risks of mortality.

A diet high in salt appears to raise our risk of high blood pressure, potentially leading to heart attacks and strokes. To boot, research has linked high salt diets to a greater risk of osteoporosis, stomach cancer, kidney disease and fluid retention.[26] As we grow older, just as we're also at greater risk of raised blood pressure, we can become more sensitive to salt and its effects.

Recently, scientists discovered that too much salt might contribute to cognitive decline and could shorten our telomeres (see page 23),[27] thereby speeding up the ageing process of our cells. Studies in mice suggest that large amounts of dietary salt can impair the microbiome, leading to impaired cognition. Salt, it seems, might be contributing to premature ageing in more ways than we originally thought.

Yet a large study published in the *Lancet* made a convincing case *for* salt. The study, which involved 130,000 people across 49 countries, found that low salt/sodium diets were associated with a greater number of heart attacks, strokes, cardiovascular disease and deaths. The authors suggested that only those with the highest salt consumption or high blood pressure need to watch their salt intake.[28]

The World Health Organization (WHO) recommends no more than 5g of salt a day (that's about a teaspoon), although the average European consumes between 7g and 18g per day, much of it from processed food; however, a recent report makes it clear that the WHO recommendations are overly cautious, finding only those people regularly consuming more than 2.5 teaspoons of table salt to be at any greater risk.[29]

Seventy-five per cent of the average daily salt intake comes from processed food, where it's effectively hidden (bread, cereals, ready meals, preserved meat, stock cubes, and so on). If you eat very little processed food and don't have high blood pressure, it's unlikely that you need to worry about your salt intake.

If your doctor has advised cutting salt, start by cooking meals from scratch. Cut out the obviously salty foods (crisps, salted nuts, bacon) but beware of some healthier foods (such as miso) which can also be very high in salt. When in doubt, check the label. Keep salt off the table and use herbs and spices to intensify the flavours of your food. Use sea salt rather than table salt (you'll find yourself using less of it and it has the benefit of a few trace minerals). Watch out for hidden salt in things such as effervescent painkillers and vitamin supplements (some can contain up to 1g of salt) and bear in mind that restaurant and takeaway food can also be very high in salt.

Our blood pressure rises as we age. As we mentioned before, recent statistics suggest one in four of us has high blood pressure without knowing it. If you haven't had your blood pressure measured recently, ask your doctor to check it (see 'Keep an Eye on Your Blood Pressure' on page 35) or invest in a home blood pressure monitor and check it yourself.

What we did:

- We swapped refined table salt for sea salt and pink Himalayan salt, which have a greater mineral content and – we think – more complex flavours.
- We keep an eye on our blood pressure.
- We replaced crisps and salty nuts with home-roasted herby nuts (see Herby Za'atar Nuts recipe on page 328).

Ditch the junk food

Where was your last meal cooked? In your kitchen, or in a factory? Half of all food bought in the UK is now considered *ultra*-processed, meaning it was made in a factory, with industrial ingredients and additives, a long way from the fresh ingredients used to cook a meal from scratch. If you cook an apple with sugar, for example, it becomes processed. But if you add emulsifiers, texturising agents and colourants, then it's ultra-processed. Britain leads Europe in our consumption of junk foods – not a race we want to win. In Portugal, just 10 per cent of food bought is ultra-processed: super-refined, packed with chemicals, oil, salt, fat and often sugar.

The European league table of junk food consumption was put together by a team of academics from across the globe. In an interview, one of the researchers – Jean-Claude Moubarac, Professor of Nutrition at the University of Montreal in Canada – said they found that ultra-processed foods:

> have very low nutritional quality in terms of the amount of free sugars, sodium [salt] and saturated fat they contain and they tend to be much lower in proteins, minerals and vita-mins ... When we compare ultra-processed foods to the rest we see striking differences [in nutritional quality]. We are recommending people limit or avoid ultra-processed foods.

The researchers also found a clear link between the amount of ultra-processed food eaten, and obesity rates: the more junk – the more obesity. Obesity is one of the highest risk factors for a wide range of degenerative diseases and chronic conditions including cancer. The World Cancer Research Fund says 'a third of the most common neoplasms [a new and abnormal growth in a tissue in the body] could be avoided by changing lifestyle and dietary habits in developed countries'.

Researchers in France have investigated the direct correlation between ultra-processed food consumption and cancer.[30] They found that for every extra 10 per cent of junk food eaten, cancer risk increases by at least 10 per cent. They don't know what causes this link. Does eating junk food mean less opportunity to eat more nutrient-dense food? Or is an additive – possibly in the packaging – causing cancer? Or is the heating process creating a carcinogenic compound? The same team is now studying food additives, and we hope that their results will shed further light on the link between junk food and cancer.

Ultra-processed food: we say

- Junk the junk. It might be cheap and tasty, but so are vegetables.
- Read the label. If you don't understand what the ingredients are, don't buy it.
- Make time to cook. All the recipes in this book (and on our blog) are simple, quick, and use minimally processed ingredients.

Refined carbohydrates – avoid, avoid, avoid (most of the time)

It's ironic that many of us who are now in mid-life, and beyond, grew up in an era when fat was considered the enemy, although it was fine to eat a huge bowl of white pasta. Experts now believe our Western epidemic of chronic lifestyle-related diseases might be a direct result of this misguided advice.

We've now cut out almost all refined carbohydrate from of our diets. This means no more heavily processed grains (like white bread, pasta and rice) in our larders. When grains are milled, they lose much of their fibre and nutritional value. The heavy processing also makes them easier to overeat, meaning we miss out on an opportunity to consume something more nutritious.

In addition, our own bodies process these foods too quickly. With no fibre to slow the digestion, they're rapidly converted from carbohydrate to glucose. There's not a lot of difference – in digestion terms – between eating sugar and eating white pasta. Once the glucose enters our blood, our bodies release insulin to keep blood sugar levels on an even keel. The insulin causes blood sugar levels to drop, so we feel hungry, and the roller-coaster starts again. Increasingly, the result is type-2 diabetes: the body fails to cope with surging insulin levels, or doesn't produce enough insulin to maintain normal glucose levels.

This is not to say that we are anti-carbohydrate, or promoting a low-carb diet. Far from it. We love unrefined, whole grains for the fibre, vitamins and health benefits they provide. A diet high in whole grains protects against type-2 diabetes, and heart and circulatory diseases. Eating a portion (28g) of whole grains a day has been associated with a 5 per cent lower risk of death from all causes and a 9 per cent lower risk of death from cardiovascular disease.[31] Another study showed that overweight adults who swapped refined grains for whole ones lost weight, ate less and reduced inflammation.[32]

Scandinavian research involving 55,000 people revealed that the type of whole grain consumed is irrelevant: they all offer protection against type-2 diabetes. The important factor is the quantity. In the study, participants eating at least 50g of whole grains daily (roughly equivalent to a bowl of porridge and a slice of rye bread) had the lowest risk of type-2 diabetes: 34 per cent lower for men and 22 per cent lower for women.[33] Recent research explains why this happens on a molecular level: whole grains increase the levels of betaine compounds in the body, which are associated with better glucose control.[34]

Our favourite whole grains

Amaranth is gluten-free, and high in protein and calcium compared to other grains. Cook like rice and throw into salads to make a complete meal.

Farro is unprocessed wheat grain, high in fibre and B vitamins. It makes a great substitute for rice or pasta.

Freekah Farro's younger, smoky cousin, freekah is unripened wheat, harvested by smoking the chaff to release the grain, which gives it a terrific flavour. It makes a fantastic salad.

Buckwheat Not wheat at all, this seed helps to control blood sugar and is high in fibre. Rinse, then soak it overnight to make a breakfast bowl; toast it and add to salads; use the flour for pancakes.

Oats Our favourite grain, oats are the most used ingredient in the recipes on our blog. Soak them in milk overnight to make a quick breakfast, or cook them for porridge. Grind them up to make flour for pancakes and cookies.

Rye helps keep blood sugar stable and is packed with magnesium. Use rye flour for pancakes and pastry.

Brown rice Packed with B vitamins, brown basmati rice is good for curries and pilaffs, and you can use short grain brown rice for risottos.

Barley Seek out pot barley rather than pearl, which has been processed. Use it to make a delicious risotto. It will take longer to cook than rice, but it's worth it.

Quinoa Really a seed, quinoa is a complete protein and contains all nine essential amino acids. Cook it like rice or grind it up to make a rough flour.

Carbohydrates: we say

- Socialising and spending time with others is as important as monitoring every morsel, so enjoy an occasional slice of cake or bowl of white pasta in good company.
- Our diets contain a wide range of whole grains for the fibre and nutrients they provide – experiment with some new ones.
- Make simple swaps: brown rice and pasta for white; wholemeal or rye bread, and not too much.
- We sit behind desks most of the day, so we don't have the same calorie requirements as our ancestors who toiled in the fields. They needed lots of carbs to keep going – we don't.
- Focus on the vegetables and good-quality protein on your plate, not the carbs.

Don't bring home the bacon (except occasionally)

We used to like a bacon sarnie or plate of ham as much as the next person, but since we started our Age-Well Project we've read too many reports linking processed meat to degenerative disease. There's a correlation between the amount of processed meat eaten and cancer risk:

- Research links high processed-meat consumption to increased oesophageal and pancreatic cancers.[35]
- An analysis of the UK Biobank (a population study of Brits aged 40–69) linked eating processed meat to breast cancer.[36]
- Every 50g of processed meat consumed daily (that's a single hot dog or two slices of bacon) was linked to a 16 per cent increased risk of bowel cancer by the American Institute of Cancer Research.[37]

The bad news doesn't stop there. A Swedish study of 37,000 men, over 12 years, found that those eating over 75g of processed meat a day were twice as likely to die of heart failure compared to those eating less than 25g. The author suggests the additives (sodium, nitrates and phosphates) are to blame.[38] Other researchers have linked the chemicals used to process red meat to an increased risk of type-2 diabetes.[39]

The World Health Organization puts processed meat in the same carcinogenic category as cigarettes and alcohol, claiming that 50g of processed meat a day raises the risk of bowel cancer by 18 per cent. But before you think that eating a sausage is tantamount to writing a suicide note, take a look at the statistics. The WHO report comes from its International Agency for

Research on Cancer (IARC). This body evaluates the strength of evidence for a substance (cigarette smoke, sunlight, sausages, for example) being carcinogenic. The report says that the evidence of a link between processed meat and cancer is as strong as the evidence of a link between smoking and cancer. It doesn't say that the risk of processed meat causing cancer is as *strong* as the risk of smoking causing cancer.

An 18 per cent increased risk of bowel cancer has to be seen in context. The chance of developing bowel cancer is 4.5 per cent across a lifetime – so a couple of rashers of bacon a day raises that risk to 5.3 per cent. It's an increase, but not a reason to give up the occasional fry-up, or slice of acorn-fed Iberico, if that's what you love. It's all a question of moderation. It's also worth considering your genes: if you have a family history of bowel cancer, you might want to reassess.

Processed meat: we say

- By 'processed meat' we mean bacon, sausages, ham and 'deli meats', such as salami and prosciutto. These are red meats – beef and, particularly, pork – that are preserved using salt, nitrates, phosphates and other additives.
- Think about how much processed meat you're eating. We eat very little now. Yes, it tastes good, but why not save it for high days and holidays?
- If you're desperately craving sausages, bacon or salami – buy the best you can.
- Use it sparingly: a crisp bacon rasher chopped and sprinkled over a salad or scrambled egg provides the taste

and texture of bacon without the need to wolf down an
entire packet.

- What can you add to your cooking to mimic the smoky
taste of bacon and sausage? We like sweet smoked paprika
or a sprinkling of smoked salt.
- Be creative with breakfast in other ways. Can you add
vegetables? Try mashed avocado on toast or sautéed
spinach with an egg.
- If your processed meat craving is a lunchtime platter of
salami and prosciutto, try some vegetarian substitutes:
sun-dried tomatoes, hummus and baba ganoush are
deliciously savoury and will simultaneously increase your
daily vegetable intake.
- Alternatively, treat yourself on your birthday, or when
you eat out.

Reduce sugar

If you're serious about ageing well you need to keep your sugar
consumption low. Early in our Age-Well Project we realised the
sweet stuff had to be drastically reduced. Our wake-up call was
a World Health Organization recommendation to halve average
sugar intake to six teaspoons (25g) a day. That's not much considering refined sugar is in almost every processed food, from
bread to soup to pasta sauce.

We know that too much sugar leads to weight gain. Refined
sugar contains nothing but calories, so our bodies use valuable
nutrients digesting it. As we age, we need fewer calories – around

1,800 a day for a 50-year-old woman – so why waste them on foods with no nutritional value?

Beyond the calories, there's increasing evidence that too much sugar consumption has a negative impact on how the body functions. In his book *The Case Against Sugar*, US journalist Gary Taubes argues that sugar has 'a unique physiological, metabolic and endocrinological (hormonal) effect on our bodies'. This effect triggers a genetic pre-disposition to obesity, above and beyond the sugar's calorific value. Taubes believes sugar is at the root of all 'the diseases of Westernization', including cancer and Alzheimer's. Not everyone agrees. Professor Michael Hornberger, Director of Ageing at Norwich Medical School, told us, 'it's not sugar but portion control that's the issue, there's nothing wrong with a small slice of home-made cake'. Other experts suspect it's the combination of low-quality carbs, fat and sugar found in junk food.

Sugar became a huge part of people's lives post-war, particularly when rising rates of heart disease were blamed on saturated fat, leading to an explosion of 'low-fat' foods. Sugar replaced fat to make these products palatable.

In recent years it's become clear that there's a correlation between sugar and heart disease. High sugar intake leads to the formation of advanced glycation end-products (AGEs) in the body, as we saw on page 22.[40] These play a key role in the development of cardiovascular disease by increasing plaque formation in the arteries.[41]

Our delicately balanced microbiomes are programmed to respond to the food we eat. Digestion starts in our mouths with saliva and the chewing process. Then, in theory, the well-chewed food makes its way into the gut where hormones are released to aid its breakdown. The gall bladder releases bile, which tells the microbiome to prepare for digestion.[42] But when we drink calorific fizzy drinks, and eat vast amounts of refined carbs, our microbiome can't prepare in time, leading to gut dysbiosis, where bad bacteria proliferates.

Recent research has linked sugar intake, and insulin levels, to cancer. Insulin appears to activate the signalling pathway known as PI3-kinase: the trigger for many cancers. Lewis Cantley, director of the Cancer Center at Weill Cornell Medicine in the US says, 'If you follow the logic that anything that drives activation of PI3-kinase ultimately results in cancer, and that insulin is the best way to do it, then that suggests that having high levels of insulin is likely to drive your cancer. And what drives insulin levels is sugar.'[43]

Sugar: we say

- Know your sugars: anything ending in '-ose' on a list of ingredients is essentially sugar. Look out for sucrose, fructose and glucose, and avoid.
- When looking at food labels, look at the total sugars. Different sugars are listed separately in ingredients, but they all add up ... to sugar!
- Over the years we've experimented with various sugar substitutes which claim to be healthier than refined sugar, such as agave syrup, stevia and xylitol. We've concluded that none of them are much better than plain sugar.
- There are a couple of exceptions: we love maple syrup, which contains antioxidants and small amounts of manganese and zinc. But it's expensive, and it's still sugar,

so we use it sparingly. Raw, unpasteurised honey contains probiotics, antioxidants and is anti-bacterial. Again, use sparingly.

- We still use sugar. We like to bake for our families, but we invariably reduce the sugar when we follow a recipe.

Cooking methods

It's not just what we cook, but how we cook that helps us age well. We've adapted some of our cooking methods as part of this project – but rest assured the changes are simple and delicious!

Fried food is high in toxic AGEs. A combination of sugars and proteins, AGEs can be created in our bodies when we eat too much sugar and refined carbohydrate. They're also formed when food is fried or grilled for a long time at a high temperature: the higher the cooking temperature, the higher the AGE content. They proliferate when food is pasteurised, dried or smoked. AGEs increase the risk of chronic disease, including diabetes and heart disease. They bind to receptors which transport beta-amyloid proteins across the blood–brain barrier, contributing to the development of Alzheimer's disease. One study found a significant correlation between diets high in AGEs and Alzheimer's.[44]

Cutting the amount of fried and processed foods we eat reduces AGE consumption, lowering inflammation. A study of AGEs and inflammation divided participants into two groups: one followed their regular Western diet, high in AGEs, and the other followed an 'AGE-less diet'. Instead of grilling, frying or baking, AGE-less foods were poached, stewed or steamed. After four months, blood AGE levels and inflammatory markers among the AGE-less group were down almost 60 per cent.[45] A similar trial of obese participants with insulin resistance found that those on the AGE-less diet showed significant improvements in insulin resistance and reduced levels of AGEs.[46]

Well-cooked meats are also a source of HCAs (heterocyclic amine compounds) formed during the cooking process. The higher the cooking temperature, and the longer the cooking time, the more HCAs are formed. Numerous studies have linked HCAs to increased cancer risk. A meta-analysis linked a high intake of well-cooked meat to an increased risk of breast, colorectal and prostate cancers.[47]

PAHs (polycyclic aromatic hydrocarbons) have also been linked to an increased cancer risk. These are formed when meat is cooked at a high temperature over an open flame. When meat fat and juices drip onto a hot plate or fire, smoke containing PAHs sticks to the meat. PAHs can also be formed during other food preparation processes, such as smoking. There is hope for the barbecue, however: research shows that marinating barbecue meat in beer before cooking reduces the formation of HCAs and PAHs.[48]

Meat is not the only culprit: research undertaken for the BBC programme *Trust Me, I'm A Doctor* suggested that polyunsaturated oils such as sunflower or corn oil are not the best choice for frying. At high temperatures, they produce high levels of aldehydes, toxic compounds linked to an increased risk of cancer, heart disease and dementia. Ironically, saturated fats, such as coconut oil and butter – and even lard (!) – are more stable at a high temperature. If you're avoiding saturated fat, use a light olive oil (not extra virgin) or rapeseed oil.

Cooking techniques: we say

- Try our Age-Well sauté technique (page 314), for healthy and delicious cooking.
- Focus on cooking techniques such as braising, steaming and stewing that cook food in liquid, and at lower temperatures.
- If you enjoy a barbecue, marinate the meat first. Or try barbecued fish or vegetable skewers instead.

CHAPTER 4

Care For Your Gut

Here we explain how to build your microbiome. Forget the pills, use probiotic-rich food and fresh air instead.

Our unique microbiome

If you've read the section 'The Role of Your Microbiome for Good Health' on page 27, you'll already know that a diverse and well-populated microbiome is now considered critical to our health and well-being. You'll also know that this is a hugely complex area that's still not fully understood.

There's one factor that's very clear, however: each of our microbiomes is different, with unique needs and requirements. Many of these change over time depending on: where we're living; our age; what we're eating; how well we're sleeping; the amount of stress in our lives; the medications we're taking; the amount of exercise we're doing – and so on.

Fortunately, there's plenty that we can do to rebalance our

microbiome, much of it not only effective but quick, easy and painless. A study reported in *Frontiers in Aging Neuroscience* found that Alzheimer's patients (who typically have different microbiomes from the rest of us) consuming a daily glass of milk enriched with beneficial bacteria showed significant improvements in cognitive functioning after only 12 weeks. This reflects other studies showing improved learning and memory following courses of probiotics.[1]

We started our Age-Well Project determined to improve our microbiomes. After increasing our consumption of fibrous prebiotic food, we set to work introducing fresh bacteria using fermented food – food created via the controlled growth of micro-organisms. There are two types of fermented food: those containing live microbes and those that don't. We concentrated on those containing live microbes: kefir, miso, yoghurt and sauerkraut, for example. Other sources include raw honey and some unprocessed cheeses. These are not to be confused with fermented foods that don't contain live bacteria, such as sourdough bread, beer and wine.

We had a go at making our own kefir, kimchi and sauerkraut, and when we bought fermented foods we avoided products that included sweeteners or were so heavily processed any microbes were inevitably dead (such as the pasteurised sauerkraut sold in most supermarkets).

But you don't have to do this. Indeed, it turns out that simply moving to a Mediterranean diet (no kimchi, kombucha or kefir needed) can increase microbiota by 7 per cent compared to 0.5 per cent on what is usually – and appropriately – termed the SAD diet (standard American diet).[2]

This might be because the Mediterranean diet is high in polyphenols, and studies show that our microbes are particularly happy when we eat a polyphenol-rich diet. The Flemish Gut Flora Project found that people consuming dark chocolate, red wine and coffee – all particularly high in polyphenols – had better functioning microbiomes. Studies of people drinking green tea or eating blueberries (both also rich in polyphenols) have found that not only do these foods increase good bacteria but they can also suppress bad bacteria, possibly reducing risks for some cancers, including colon cancer.[3]

We can boost our microbiomes in other ways, too – it's not all about the food we eat. Professor Tim Spector, author of *The Diet Myth*, suggests the following have a beneficial impact: spending time outside; being in the country; gardening; living with – or merely stroking – a dog. His studies found marked differences between the microbiomes of rural and urban people, gardeners and non-gardeners, pet-owners (particularly those with dogs) and non-pet-owners. Professor Spector also suggests a good sleeping routine to help nurture our microbiome, following reports of disrupted sleep appearing to negatively alter populations of gut bacteria.[4]

What about probiotic supplements, though? Researchers are divided. A study published in *Genome Magazine* found that probiotic supplements (from drinks to capsules) had no effect.[5] If you're determined to take one, look for a high-potency probiotic with at least 50 million live bacteria from a variety of strains. When University College London tested eight probiotic supplements (including the obvious names), only one ever made it to – and survived in – the small intestine.[6]

Feed your microbiome: we say

- Include a fermented food in your weekly diet. A bowl of yoghurt a few times a week is fine.
- Forget commercial probiotic supplements, drinks and products.
- Eat polyphenol-rich foods every day (like berries, beans and dark chocolate).
- Get outside in the fresh air. Open the windows, stroke dogs, garden, forage or hug trees.
- Feed your microbiome with plenty of fibrous prebiotic-rich fruit, vegetables, whole grains and nuts (walnuts have been found to be very effective).[7]

Maintain your microbiome

When it comes to keeping your microbiome in good condition, it's not just about the prebiotics and the probiotics. If you've read previous sections you'll know your gut loves prebiotic fibrous plants, regular doses of probiotic-rich fermented food, and a Mediterranean diet brimming with polyphenols. But is this enough to create and sustain the gut diversity we need to age well? How else can we maintain and nurture the pulsating galaxy of bacteria living within us?

A recent study published in *Nature's Scientific Reports* analysed data from 876 middle-aged and elderly women and found that those who consumed the most omega-3 fats had the most diverse microbiomes, regardless of their prebiotic or probiotic intake. Researchers found that high levels of omega-3 correlated with a gut compound called N-carbamylglutamate, already known to reduce oxidative stress in the guts of animals. The researchers speculate that omega-3 might encourage bacteria to produce N-carbamylglutamate.[8]

The Flemish Gut Flora Project found that medication had the biggest influence on the diversity of our microbiome. Antibiotics, proton-pump inhibitors (a heartburn drug), metformin (a diabetes drug), laxatives and hay fever drugs were all linked to lower gut diversity. To keep our gut at its optimum we may need to be a little more vigilant about our use of medication. Now, when our doctors want to prescribe antibiotics for us, we ask if there's an alternative. Frequently, there is.

It isn't just medication we need to be aware of. Certain foods can also destroy our carefully rebuilt guts. The Flemish Gut Project found a correlation between lower microbiome diversity and diets high in sugar, carbohydrates, calories, whole milk and frequent snacking.[9] Cheese, however, is a different matter altogether. A small Danish study found that cheese-eaters had increased concentrations of butyrate, a compound with powerful anti-inflammatory effects that can protect against bowel cancer, among other things.[10]

How we cook has an impact on our biota too. Diets high in fried food correlate with diminished diversity, whereas diets with plenty of raw and lightly cooked food correlate with improved diversity.

Intermittent fasting or a daily period of at least 12 hours without food appears to allow the microbiome to reboot itself.[11] Small-scale studies suggest that fasting increases microbial diversity and allows a bacteria called *Akkermansia* to flourish.[12] *Akkermansia*, a strain of bacteria that often turns up in the microbiomes of long-lived people, has been associated with staying thin and avoiding diabetes. It strengthens the walls of the gut and reduces inflammation. Studies of mice suggest it can be increased by consuming fish oils – and by fasting.[13]

Surprisingly, exercise might also help us to nurture our microbiomes. We know exercise is good for our heart and brain, but new research suggests that it might be just as good for our guts. A recent study found that people who exercised altered the composition of their guts, even changing the genes of many microbes, without any changes to their diet. After six weeks of no exercise, however, their microbiomes had reverted back, so keep your exercise programme going.[14]

What about our love of cleanliness? Jeff Leach, founder of American Gut, urges us to worry less about germs and to be less rigorous with hand sanitisers and home cleaning products. A slightly less hygienic environment might, he suggests, be beneficial for our biomes.

Lastly, regular sleep patterns appear to benefit our microbiome. Certain strains of gut flora, like *Lactobacillus*, seem to increase as we sleep and decrease when we're awake. Early studies on mice show that disrupted sleep leads to a disrupted microbiome, and researchers have suggested that our microbiota might have their own circadian rhythms.[15]

Nurture your microbiome: we say

- Think before you reach for the antibiotics (but always discuss this with your GP).
- Eat a diet rich in plants, fermented foods and omega-3s.
- Aim for as much variety as possible, ideally 30 plants a week.

- Replace fried foods with steamed, raw or sautéed.
- Keep exercising.
- Fast between meals with a 12-hour daily break between supper and breakfast.
- Keep regular sleep patterns.
- Don't be excessively concerned with hygiene.

Some of our favourite fermented foods

Miso is an addictive, savoury paste made from fermented soya beans and, sometimes, grains. It makes a wonderful base for soups. Throw in some noodles and vegetables, and you have a healthy pot noodle, or add a little to salad dressings.

Sauerkraut This Eastern European delicacy is testament to what can be achieved with the simplest of ingredients. Made from just cabbage, salt and spices, it partners almost any savoury dish. We like it with fish.

Kimchi This Korean version of sauerkraut is made with garlic and chilli. It can be used like sauerkraut, or to top curries and stir-fries. Try it alongside poached eggs or avocado on toast for a gut-friendly breakfast. Drained and chopped finely it can be stirred into batter to make savoury pancakes, or mixed with equal quantities of Greek yoghurt and cream cheese for a rich, piquant dip.

Live yoghurt Make sure you're buying live, probiotic yoghurt. It might be a little more expensive, but it's an easy way to get some good bacteria into the whole family. Top with fresh fruit and some low-sugar granola for an invigorating start to the day.

Kefir is a cultured milk drink that's delicious on its own or in a smoothie. Pour it over fruit or granola for a snack. Professor Tim Spector, director of the British Gut Project, refers to kefir as 'super-yoghurt'.

Kombucha is a refreshing fermented tea that is available in lots of flavours. Do check the sugar content, though. Drink it chilled. Mix with vodka, lime juice and ice for a cheeky cocktail.

Fermented foods: we say

- We dislike suggesting *anything* that might add to the busy-ness of life, but fermenting your own foods is particularly satisfying. Try it and see.
- You can buy kefir grains online and, if you look after them, they constantly replenish themselves.
- Sauerkraut is easy: massage one tablespoon of salt into a finely chopped cabbage and seal in a sterilised Kilner-type jar for at least five days – and up to a month. There are lots of recipes and tips online.
- Plan how to get your regular probiotics. Some yoghurt for breakfast, a dollop of kimchi with a lunchtime salad or a kombucha drink mid-afternoon? Once you get into the habit of eating fermented foods it becomes much easier.
- Check the quality of what you're buying. Supermarket

sauerkraut is often fermented in vinegar and pasteurised, so it doesn't contain the same probiotics as naturally fermented foods.

- Too much fermented food can affect those with a compromised digestion. A spoonful of yoghurt most days is quite sufficient unless your microbiome is severely depleted. Some researchers still question exactly how many bacteria survive the journey to our intestines.

CHAPTER 5

What to Eat

When we started writing about ageing well, we focused on healthy eating, which seemed the simplest, easiest way to improve our health. In the intervening years we have expanded our knowledge in many different directions – but how we eat continues to be at the heart of everything we do. In this chapter, we cover the most significant nutrients for healthy longevity and reveal how we included them in our diets.

Eat green

We grew up to the constant refrain of 'eat your greens'. Now we repeat it endlessly to our own children. But with good reason: green vegetables are the most nutrient-dense foods on earth, packing a huge range of vitamins and minerals for very little calorie content. If we had to pick one Age-Well food, it would be green vegetables.

In a league table of 'powerhouse fruits and vegetables', ranked by nutrient density score, green leafy vegetables dominated the top 20. Watercress scored a perfect 100, closely followed by pak choi (Chinese cabbage), chard, greens, spinach, chicory and lettuce. Cruciferous (brassica) vegetables, such as kale, broccoli and Brussels sprouts weren't far behind. One-hundred grams of each of these vegetables provides at least 10 per cent of our daily requirement of key nutrients, including potassium, calcium, iron, zinc and vitamins A, B_6, B_{12}, C, D, E and K.[1]

Experts are fascinated by these green powerhouses: every year hundreds of research papers investigate how they reduce our risk of age-related chronic illness.

One study in particular had us loading our supermarket trollies with green vegetables. It suggested that eating greens might help to slow the rate of cognitive decline to that of someone 11 years younger. The study followed almost 1,000 people, aged between 58 and 99, for five years and found that the rate of cognitive decline in those eating a daily portion of leafy green vegetables was much slower than in those who ate none. The research team attributed this to the positive impact of phylloquinone, lutein and folate – all found in green vegetables – on our brains.[2]

Further evidence of the benefits of greens comes from research into heart health. Green leafy vegetables are packed with a chemical compound called nitric oxide. This keeps our artery linings smooth and well functioning. Reduced levels of nitric oxide play a part in many cardiovascular issues, including hypertension. Researchers in Japan fed mice a diet low in nitric oxide. After 18 months the mice had hypertension, insulin resistance and weight gain. After 22 months they were dying of heart disease.[3] Crucially, it's not only mice. Research from Australia revealed that women over 70 who ate three portions of cruciferous vegetables each day had a reduced risk of subclinical atherosclerosis (hardening of the arteries).[4]

Further research shows that eating green vegetables might also improve the immune system,[5] as well as reducing the risk of diabetes. A review by the University of Leicester found that a daily portion of green vegetables could reduce the risk of type-2 diabetes by 14 per cent. Glaucoma risk is reduced by as much as 30 per cent, according to a review by the Harvard School of Public Health.[6]

Finally, many green vegetables, including spinach, asparagus, Brussels sprouts and broccoli, are rich in the nutrient folate. It's a B vitamin crucial for DNA synthesis and cellular repair. It also helps us to maintain low levels of homocysteine, an amino acid produced in the body and linked (at high levels) to hardening of the arteries and shorter telomere length.[7] See Chapter 1 for more on telomeres, but the longer our telomeres, the less damage there is to our DNA and the greater our chances of healthy longevity.

Green vegetables: we say

- Include green vegetables in every meal.
- Add baby spinach to a smoothie for breakfast, have a salad for lunch and sauté kale for dinner.
- Keep vegetable purées and spinach in the freezer to throw into anything, from a smoothie to a sauce for fish.
- Think creatively with your vegetables: massage kale with a little olive oil and salt to make a salad, braise lettuce,

grate broccoli, add courgettes to cakes, roast wedges
of cabbage.
- Try foraging for wild green vegetables such as young
  nettles, dandelion leaves and wild garlic.
- Experiment with growing your own: salad vegetables can
  be grown in window boxes and pots.

Eat colourfully

When we started our Age-Well Project, we often heard the
phrase 'eat the rainbow'. We now eat a glorious array of coloured
fruit and vegetables every day: from the deep, Gothic purples of
blueberries and aubergines to the pearlescent whites of onions
and leeks.

The glowing colours of fruit and vegetables make them attractive to animals – including humans – who then disseminate the
seeds. Mother Nature is very clever when she needs something
doing, and we're rewarded for eating these beautiful natural
creations with a multitude of health benefits.

This is complicated, but in a nutshell phyto- (plant-) chemistry
works as follows. Highly coloured fruit and veg derive their pigments from carotenoids (orange, red or yellow) or polyphenols
(pretty much all the other colours). Both act as antioxidants,
fighting cell damage in the body. They may also influence gut
microbiota. Bioflavonoids, a sub-group of polyphenols, are
found in tea, honey, wine, fruits, vegetables, nuts, olive oil,
cocoa and grains. Anthocyanins, a sub-group of flavonoids, are
found in indigo/purple fruits and vegetables such as blueberries,

aubergines and blackberries. Most plants contain more than one polyphenol or carotenoid, all working in synergy. But to keep it simple we'll use colour.

Red, orange and yellow

Foods such as carrots, sweet potatoes, peppers, squash, watermelon and tomatoes get their colour from carotenoids. These sub-divide into – among other substances – beta-carotene, lycopene, lutein and betacyanins.

- Beta-carotenes are converted into retinol (the active form of vitamin A) to boost eye health and the immune system.[8]
- Lycopene gives tomatoes and watermelon their rich colour. Research has shown that this phyto-nutrient has a powerful effect on cancer, particularly prostate cancer.[9]
- Betacyanins, found in beetroot, chard stems and rhubarb, are anti-inflammatory and have been found to have a beneficial effect on liver, colon, bladder and breast cancers.[10]

Green

We talked about the power of green vegetables at the beginning of this chapter. Green vegetables get their strong colour from chlorophyll, which is at the heart of the photosynthesis process, enabling plants to absorb energy from the sun and, with the help of water, use it for their own nourishment.

- Chlorophyll absorbs red and blue light, then creates carbohydrates for the plant. It's a rich source of the anti-oxidants that protect our cells from free-radical damage.
- The darker the green vegetable, the more chlorophyll it contains, so spinach, kale and parsley are all excellent sources.

Blues and purples

These colours are created in plants such as blueberries, beetroots and cherries by flavonoids called anthocyanins:

- Research suggests that they can improve eyesight, including night vision.
- They might also reduce cancer cell growth and prevent tumours forming.
- As antioxidants, they protect against heart disease. Tests using anthocyanins extracted from elderberries demonstrated that they were able to protect endothelial cells (which line our arteries) from damage by oxidation and reduce inflammation.[11]

White

White fruits and vegetables get their pigment from polyphenols called anthoxanthins.

- Anthoxanthins might help reduce heart disease, Alzheimer's and cancer risk.
- Allicin, the active compound in fresh garlic and onions, is antibacterial and anti-fungal. It might also help to lower

the risk of high blood pressure and high cholesterol.[12] It also helps with the management of type-2 diabetes.[13]

- Onions also contain a flavonoid called quercetin. Research suggests that it's anti-inflammatory and helps to support respiratory health.

Researchers haven't yet uncovered how the process works or quite how each pigment interacts with the others, or with our bodies, so there's no agreed 'dose' of polyphenols or carotenoids.[14] We've added a wide variety of highly coloured fruit and veg to our Age-Well diets to make sure we get to the end of the rainbow!

Eating the rainbow: we say

- Think 'colour' in the supermarket or greengrocers. What can you pick up in your weekly shop that's going to add colour to your plate?
- Consider a weekly organic vegetable box or bag. You'll get an array of seasonal produce, and if it's already in the house, you're more likely to use it.
- Pack your plate with colour.
- Try spending an hour each week meal prepping. Roast a tray of vegetables, prepare some crudités, make a couple of brightly coloured, vegetable-based dips or sauces. These can be stored in the fridge for an instant rainbow meal.
- Experiment with new recipes using colourful fruit and vegetables.

• Keep a bowl or freezer bag of pre-chopped vegetables –
  peppers, carrot sticks, cucumber – in the fridge for
  snacking or dipping.

Know your omegas

When scientists refer to a group of nutrients as essential, you
know it's time to pay attention. Essential fatty acids (EFAs)
are nutrients that our bodies can't manufacture, so we have to
ingest them from food or supplements. EFAs fall into two main
categories: omega-6s and omega-3s.[15] We're born with a supply
that dwindles as we age: hence the need to consume enough to
keep us healthy.

These polyunsaturated fats play a critical role in the function
of every cell in our bodies. They form a key part of our cell
membranes, regulating neurotransmitters (the brain's messaging
service), insulin function and inflammation. Recent research
revealed that older adults with higher circulating levels of EFAs
were nearly 20 per cent less likely to be suffering a chronic ageing
disease like cardiovascular disease or cancer.[16]

An analysis of data from 19 different studies involving more
than 45,000 people from 16 countries found that those with higher
levels of omega-3 in their blood were 10 per cent less likely to die
from a heart attack than those with lower concentrations.[17] Omega-
3s also reduce inflammation in the body and have been linked to
better gut health. Research from the University of Nottingham
found that omega-3 intake was 'strongly associated with the diversity and number of species of healthy bacteria in the gut'.[18]

Our brains are 60 per cent fatty acid, made up of docosahexaenoic acid (DHA) and eicosapentaenoic acid (EPA), both omega-3 fats. They coat our brain cells, protecting them from injury and inflammation. Declining DHA and EPA as we age leaves us vulnerable to memory loss, mood disorders, reduced brain volume and Alzheimer's.

A study assessed the omega-3 consumption of older adults with the ApoE4 gene (and therefore at risk of late-onset Alzheimer's). Those who consumed more omega-3 fatty acids had better cognitive flexibility, the ability to efficiently switch between tasks.[19] The lead scientist said, 'Recent research suggests a critical link between nutritional deficiencies and the incidence of both cognitive impairment and degenerative neurological disorders, such as Alzheimer's. Our findings add to the evidence that optimal nutrition helps preserve cognitive function, slow the progression of ageing and reduce the incidence of debilitating diseases.'

If we consume lots of omega-3, therefore, we'll live to a ripe old age? Unfortunately it's not that simple. Research shows that the balance of omega-3 fatty acids to other fatty acids, particularly omega-6, is critical. Omega-6 is freely available in the Western diet: it's found in fried foods, processed oils and factory-farmed meat. Our omega-6 to omega-3 ratio should be between 4:1 and 2:1, but, in the West, average ratios are around 15:1.

The ratio of omega-3 to omega-6 has a fundamental effect on one of the key markers of healthy ageing: our telomeres. These are the vital caps that protect our DNA from damage as we age. A double-blind study of middle-aged and older overweight, sedentary adults found supplementing with omega-3 to alter the ratio of fatty acid consumption protected telomeres.[20] When the researchers analysed the ratio of omega-3 to -6, they found the lower the ratio, the longer the telomeres.

How, then, do we redress the balance? There's no exact definition of what the balance of omega-3 and omega-6 should be, and no recommended daily allowance (RDA) of either. To reduce our levels of omega-6 we've cut our intake of processed food, factory-farmed meats and seed oils such as sunflower and corn oil. To increase our omega-3 levels we eat two portions of oily fish and a few eggs each week. We get ALA, a plant-based omega-3, from walnuts, chia seeds and flax seeds.

If you don't eat fish, the liver can convert ALA to EPA and then to DHA, but this process isn't very efficient – only around 15 per cent of ALA ends up as DHA.[21] As research director Professor Minihane told us, 'Plant-based omega-3s are difficult for the liver to convert unless you're a pre-menopausal female. Oddly, vegans and red wine drinkers often have higher levels of DHA suggesting a polyphenol may be acting synergistically with another compound or that a plant-based diet might be assisting the liver in some way.'[22]

Essential fatty acids: we say

- Read the next section on oily fish for the benefits and sustainability of fish-sourced DHA and EPA.
- We eat two portions of oily fish a week: salmon, mackerel, herrings and anchovies are all good sources. We're particularly partial to tinned sardines: cheap, sustainable and convenient.
- Nuts are a rich source of ALA, 30g of walnuts contains 2.6g

ALA. In the US, the National Institutes of Health suggests an 'adequate daily intake' of 1.6g of ALA for men and 1.1g for women.

- Sprinkle walnuts on salads or use instead of pine nuts in a home-made pesto.
- Chia seeds are probably the best plant-based source of ALA with 1 tablespoon (15g) providing 2.7g. Add a spoonful to overnight oats, layer soaked chia seeds with yoghurt and fruit for a dessert or buy them ready ground and use in baking.
- Flax seeds can also be bought ready ground – substitute a tablespoon for flour in pancakes or biscuits for an omega-3 boost.
- Note: the humble pea contains ALA.
- One of the many benefits of fermentation is its ability to produce omega-3s. Read more about fermented foods in Chapter 4.
- Consider marine algae supplements if you're vegan or vegetarian.

Oily fish

Oily fish – cold-water fish containing high levels of omega-3 fatty acids – have become synonymous with healthy eating. The trend for eating more oily fish started in the 1970s when researchers in Greenland realised the Inuit (whose diet is rich in oily fish) had a very low instance of heart disease.[23] Since then, consumption of oily fish has been linked to a lower risk of many cancers, asthma, diabetes, high blood pressure, macular degeneration, MS, dementia and rheumatoid arthritis. A review of data from nearly half a million people found that those who ate the most oily fish were less likely to die, from any cause, than those who ate the least, while women who ate plenty of oily fish were found to have a 38 per cent reduced chance of dying from Alzheimer's.[24]

Cold-water fish need extra fat to keep their muscles flexible. They consume marine algae, rich in omega-3s, and concentrate it in their cells so that they can continue swimming in freezing seas. The power of oily fish comes from its docosahexaenoic acid (DHA), an omega-3 fatty acid that our bodies can't make by themselves. It's vital to the structure of our cell membranes, keeping them flexible and strong. As we saw earlier, our brains are 60 per cent fatty acids, up to 90 per cent of which is DHA. As we age, our supplies of DHA dwindle, and we can't make more without the right nutrition. Oily fish is the richest source on the planet.

After reading research showing people who regularly ate salmon had lower incidences of dementia, oily fish became a vital component of our Age-Well diet. The same report also investigated whether fish eaters had higher levels of mercury in their brains. They didn't.[25] But we still had concerns about the chemicals used in salmon farming and the environmental impact of both sea fishing and intensive fish farming. Headlines such as 'Farmed salmon has more fat than pizza' didn't help.[26]

Farmed salmon is a great source of omega-3 fatty acid: in fact, it has more per gram than wild salmon; however, it can also have nearly six times as much omega-6. If you've read the previous section on 'Know Your Omegas' you'll know how important it is to balance omega-3 and omega-6. So, although we occasionally eat farmed salmon (organic where possible), we typically look elsewhere for our omega-3s. Eating a wide range of fish is also important. Professor Minihane has carried out extensive research into oily fish and told us that she eats three portions of fish a week, 'an oily fish, a white fish and perhaps a shellfish. Diversity is really important.' She also takes a daily omega-3 supplement.

We love experimenting with wild-caught, sustainable fish such as anchovies, mackerel (fresh or smoked), trout, sardines, pilchards and herring. These smaller fish are far enough down the food chain to be lower in mercury and other pollutants than bigger fish such as tuna. We're great fans of tinned sardines: not the fancy ones in beautiful tins, but the cheap and cheerful own-brand sardines. Average price? Forty pence a can. These nutritional powerhouses are high in omega-3s and calcium, while containing virtually no mercury. They also contain iron, magnesium, phosphorus, potassium, zinc, copper, selenium and manganese, as well as a full complement of B vitamins. Don't buy the filleted sardines – the bones are packed with calcium.

If you dislike the taste of fish, try slipping a few anchovies into a meat stew or a tin of sardines into a garlicky tomato sauce for pouring over pasta.

Oily fish: we say

- There's no need to overeat oily fish – two portions a week is enough.
- Try mashing sardines (bones and all) with a little butter and spreading on toast for a quick lunch.
- Fried fish doesn't count – sorry! The researchers who

found eating fish reduces the risk of death, also found that eating fried fish brings no benefits. Perhaps because frying creates trans fats and adds calories.

- Oily fish with a high DHA content include: salmon, sardines, halibut, scallops, shrimp, anchovies, herring, mackerel, pilchards, trout, fresh tuna, crab and whitebait.
- Jars of pickled herrings make a good store-cupboard standby.
- Look out for the Marine Stewardship Council's blue label, which certifies fish coming from a sustainable source. Ask your fishmonger if in doubt.

Why we eat pulses every day

It's rare to find a list of longevity-boosting foods that doesn't include pulses, also known as legumes (peas, beans and lentils) in the top ten. Lentils and beans are a mainstay of the Mediterranean diet, widely recognised as the most effective way of eating to reduce age-related degenerative diseases.

Dan Buettner, who researches Blue Zones (the areas of the world with the highest concentrations of centenarians), describes pulses as 'the world's greatest longevity food'. Apparently the average Blue Zoner eats a cup of beans a day – be that edamame (soya) beans in Japan's Okinawa or cannellini beans in Sardinia.

Why, then, do these humble foods earn all the plaudits?

They're packed with protein, fibre, vitamins and minerals: 100g of cooked lentils provides around 9g of protein and 8g of fibre. This means we feel fuller for longer: studies have linked pulses to weight loss. As a low-glycaemic food they also help to stabilise blood sugar.

They are rich in antioxidants Research from China revealed high levels of polyphenols in all beans and pulses (and lentils in particular). Polyphenols are powerful tools in the fight against diabetes, obesity, heart disease, cancer and inflammation.[27, 28]

They reduce the risk of diabetes Clinical studies show that the consumption of three or more servings of beans a week reduces the risk of diabetes by almost 35 per cent.[29] In a small study, sufferers of metabolic syndrome (often a precursor to type-2 diabetes and heart disease) who ate black beans every day showed increased insulin sensitivity, leading the researchers to conclude that regular consumption of black beans could delay the onset of cardiovascular disease and type-2 diabetes.[30]

They lower blood pressure One study found that eating about 190g (1 cup/250ml by volume) of legumes a day could reduce the risk of coronary heart disease by lowering blood pressure.[31]

They improve cholesterol levels Another study found that eating pulses significantly reduced levels of LDL – aka 'bad' cholesterol in the blood. High levels of LDL are linked to heart disease.[32]

Better cancer outcomes A Spanish study linked consumption of legumes to a reduced risk of death from cancer.[33]

Good gut health Pulses contain prebiotics, boosting our microbiota. Good gut health appears to help fend off many age-related diseases and conditions, from cancer and Alzheimer's to arthritis.

Pulses: we say

- Eat lentils and beans most days: chickpeas, kidney beans, cannellini beans, black beans, haricot beans, butter beans, black-eyed peas, and red, green and brown lentils.
- Stock up on a wide variety – vacuum packed, tinned and dried – and be creative. Add pulses to casseroles, blend them into dips or sprinkle them over salads.
- Use defrosted edamame (soya) beans in stir-fries or grain bowls.
- Put pulses in puddings: whizz chickpeas into cookie recipes or try dessert hummus: blend a drained and rinsed tin of chickpeas, 2 tablespoons nut butter, cocoa or raw cacao, a little maple syrup and a dash of water and use as a dip for sliced fruits.
- Use a handful of small red lentils to add density to soups.
- Plan a meal around a pulse. Italian bean stew and black bean tacos are popular in our households.
- Swap mashed potato for mashed butter beans. Add a little olive oil, chopped fresh rosemary and season well.
- Sprouted pulses are delicious and full of nutrients. Try growing your own or buy ready-sprouted.

Tuck into guilt-free cheese

We cheered after a report appeared suggesting that regular cheese eaters live longer, healthier lives. Announced at the 2018

European Society of Cardiology Congress, a 15-year study of over 636,000 people found that eating cheese was associated with an 8 per cent lower total mortality risk. We were vindicated: for years we'd argued on our blog that cheese was being demonised. Instead of shunning cheese for its fat content, we maintained that good cheese was essential to ageing well, not to mention having an enjoyable old age. After all, cheese played a crucial role in the diets of our ancestors and is regularly consumed in many Blue Zones.

That's all changed now, particularly in the light of a second study confirming the protective effects of cheese on the heart. Researchers speculate that the arrangement of protein and calcium might hold the answers, given that the same benefits aren't accorded to milk or butter.

We're not suggesting everyone eats from a vast cheeseboard every day. Instead, we're asking people to invest a little bit more and eat real cheese. Because it's in real cheese that we find the flavours, nutrients (like spermidine) and bacteria that make it a truly life-enhancing food. Real cheese incidentally is cheese made the old-fashioned way on farms, not in factories. It never comes as a plastic-wrapped slice or – God forbid – a string.

Several other reports now attest to the extraordinary properties of cheese. A small Danish study compared the diet of the French (average annual cheese consumption: 23.9kg) with that of the British (average annual cheese consumption: 11.6kg). The French typically have longer life expectancy, lower rates of cardiovascular disease – still the leading cause of premature death in the UK – and far less obesity, so does the secret lie in their hefty appetite for cheese? The researchers certainly thought so, explaining that cheese contains butyric acid, a short-chain fatty acid thought to have anti-inflammatory powers, as well as cell and gut-healing properties.[34]

This so-called French paradox was also explored by Professor Tim Spector as he researched his book, *The Diet Myth*. 'If eating saturated fat is so bad,' he asked, 'why do the French ... suffer from less than a third the rate of heart disease as the Brits?' To find out, he ate 180g of French cheese, daily, for three days. He collected and analysed his stool samples and found – in a single day – significant changes to his microbiota. In particular he noted substantial increases in the quantity of *Lactobacilli* (a protective bacterium that lines the intestines). These lasted for the duration of his cheese diet, returning to their usual levels once he stopped eating cheese.

It isn't only the French that benefit from a generous cheese consumption. The Swiss, one of the longest-living populations in the world, eat an average of 21.3kg of cheese a year. Much of this, unsurprisingly, is Swiss cheese such as Gruyère and Emmental – both of which also happen to contain the only natural source of an essential strain of gut bacteria known as *Propionibacterium freudenreichii*. This bacteria releases propionic acid, the favourite food of all seven strains of another gut bacteria called bifidobacteria. In one study, people eating 100g of Swiss cheese a day for two weeks increased their bifidobacteria levels by 800 per cent, while a study last year found that consuming *Propionibacterium freudenreichii* increased the life span of worms, prompting the researchers to suggest that this particular strain might somehow trigger an anti-inflammatory response in the body.[35]

Other researchers have speculated that cheese's miracle ingredient could be alkaline phosphatase, an anti-inflammatory enzyme found in blue cheese and raw milk products.[36] This might explain the famed longevity in the cheese-loving Blue Zones of Sardinia and Ikaria. In Sardinia (known as 'home to the longest-living men'), when asked what they attributed their longevity to, the inhabitants famously replied 'wine and the local pecorino cheese'. On the Greek island of Ikaria, a raw Feta-style goat's cheese is liberally eaten.[37]

Of course, cheese is also a good source of vitamins A, D and B (in particular B_{12} and folate, both essential for methylation – a biochemical process that helps regulate how the body detoxifies itself, among other things, protein, zinc, magnesium and calcium. We lose bone density from our mid-thirties, and without an adequate supply of calcium we risk getting osteoporosis in old age – another good reason to eat a little cheese every now and then.

Later in the book we explore the intriguing longevity-enhancing properties of spermidine, a nutrient found in aged and blue cheeses such as French Roquefort. Spermidine has been linked to a reduced risk of liver cancer, lower blood pressure, better heart health and a longer lifespan.[38]

- Seek out local cheeses, remembering that those made from raw/unpasteurised milk will have more probiotic content and more alkaline phosphatase (note: raw milk is not recommended for those with compromised immune systems).
- A slither of the best cheese you can afford will always be more satisfying than a lump of cheap processed cheese.
- Of particular note for their health benefits are: blue cheeses, Swiss cheeses such as Gruyère and Emmental, and the Feta and Parmesan enjoyed by the long-lived Ikarian and Sardinian Blue Zoners.
- Don't gorge. Most cheese is still high in fat and sodium.
- Eat alongside a green salad and some fruit.

Cheer up with ... chocolate

The case for chocolate is stronger than ever: chocolate might actually keep you young. But only the right type.

Over the last decade, an outpouring of research has suggested that chocolate can reduce stress and inflammation, improve memory, immunity and mood, reduce the risk of diabetes, stroke and heart disease, lower the chance of an irregular heartbeat, help beat migraines, improve cardiovascular health, lower blood pressure and 'bad' cholesterol, reduce the risk of colon cancer, strengthen cell membranes, protect against liver damage and disease, and prevent the formation of blood clots.

A small but interesting 2018 study found that regularly consuming dark chocolate increased the expression of genes involved in activating T-cells (the white blood cells that fight infection and disease) as well as the genes involved in neural signalling (the transmission of information between neurons). The same study also found that the higher the concentration of cacao the greater the impact on cognition, mood, immunity and memory.[39] In other words, chocolate is good for both the brain and the body. Indeed, chocolate appears to be a veritable elixir of health, youth and vitality.[40]

Not, however, the chocolate bars that typically line our supermarket shelves. The research listed above is based entirely on very dark chocolate, containing over 70 per cent cacao. Many studies show that the darker the chocolate, the greater the health benefits, so it's worth cultivating a palate for chocolate with the highest possible cacao content.

Experts still don't know why dark chocolate has such extraordinary benefits. It might be because the flavanols in cacao help blood flow around the body and to the brain.

It might be because cacao is a great source of antioxidants, protecting our cells from damage and inflammation. On the ORAC scale (the measure used by scientists to determine the antioxidant content of food), raw cacao beans are among the highest scoring foods ever tested. In particular, experts have drawn attention to a flavanol called epicatechin, present in particularly high doses in cacao.

Cacao also contains valeric acid, a stress reducer, as well as the stimulants caffeine and theobromine – making it simultaneously soothing and stimulating. In addition to all these, it contains an arsenal of other nutrients, including iron, calcium, zinc, phosphorus and magnesium.

How much chocolate can we eat each day? Many of the trials above used small 40–55g bars, while some used cocoa – in which case experts advise mixing it with low-fat milk or water. We think that sounds a little unappetising, so we usually tuck into a few small squares – as do two of Europe's leading chocolate researchers[41] – and don't worry too much about the fat and sugar content, which is typically less the darker the chocolate. Apparently 40g of dark chocolate is ideal.[42]

More important than asking how much, however, is asking what sort. Look at the percentage of cocoa solids listed on the label and aim for anything above 70 per cent. We prefer 85 per cent, but that's only after a few years of slowly reducing our sugar consumption. To acclimatise your palate start at around 50 per cent cocoa solids and move up as your taste buds adjust.

Flavanol content varies wildly from brand to brand and even from batch to batch, depending in part on the temperature at which the beans have been roasted. Raw chocolate, however, can't be heated above 45°C, which suggests it might more effectively preserve flavanol content and other phytonutrients. We particularly like Pacari, whose award-winning raw, organic chocolate bar regularly beats off competition from traditional chocolatiers.

If you're watching your fat and sugar intake, opt for drinking unsweetened cocoa, which has 88–96 per cent cocoa solids, but none of the downsides.

Cacao crops are often heavily sprayed. We'd suggest opting for organic if and when you can.

- Enjoy dark chocolate with a minimum of 70 per cent cocoa solids.
- Choose organic and/or raw, if you like it and you can.
- Eat it in moderation, as with all things. We like 3–4 squares with a cup of tea.

Healthy spermidine – why we love wheatgerm

Spermidine is the rather unfortunate name for a polyamine first discovered in – yes, you guessed it – human semen. Since then it's been found in most human tissue and in all organisms from bacteria to mammals and humans. More importantly, spermidine has caused great excitement among the group of scientists who've been investigating its extraordinary age-enhancing powers.

During the last decade, spermidine has been found to extend the healthy life of fruit flies, yeast, worms and rodents. Spermidine supplements have resulted in: reduced rates of liver fibrosis and cancerous liver tumours;[43] improved heart health;[44] reduced rates of age-related cognitive and motor impairment;[45] and reduced inflammation and oxidative stress.[46] In some animals spermidine has resulted in extending life by as much as 25 per cent.

More recently research has begun on humans. Early results look promising, with studies suggesting people on spermidine-rich diets have lower blood pressure, and lower rates of both cardiovascular disease and stroke.[47] A recent study in the *American Journal of Clinical Nutrition* found a difference of 5.7 years between those on the lowest and highest spermidine-containing diets, suggesting that spermidine might indeed play a role in longevity.[48] Mediterranean diets are thought to contain almost twice as much spermidine as those typically eaten in Northern Europe and America. Could this be why those on a Mediterranean diet have better health? Research continues, and we wouldn't recommend taking spermidine supplements (indeed at the time of writing there are no over-the-counter spermidine supplements that we know of).

Scientists still don't fully understand quite how or why spermidine works, but it appears that spermidine induces autophagy (the process by which cells clear out accumulating debris), making it an alternative to caloric restriction, which works in the same way. Many scientists refer to spermidine, for this reason, as a caloric restriction mimetic.

Spermidine can be adequately sourced through a healthy diet and appears fairly safe. As Dr Rafael de Cabo, a scientist at the US Institute on Aging, said, 'It could be relatively easy for most people to get the benefits of spermidine through dietary modifications.'

We researched sources of spermidine and found it present in many of our favourite ingredients: blue cheese, hard fermented cheeses such as Cheddar, Gruyère, Parmesan or Manchego, peas, soya beans, lentils, mushrooms, miso, pears, broccoli, cauliflower and leafy greens. It's also in most meat: according to the Swedish Karolinska Institute, meat and vegetables contain the highest spermidine content. But the richest source of spermidine is actually ... wheatgerm. While blue cheese contains an average of 262nmol (nanomoles) per gram and peas 173nmol per gram, wheatgerm contains a whopping 2,440nmol per gram. Researchers devising trials of spermidine typically use wheatgerm, the nutrient-dense centre of a wheat kernel.

Wheatgerm also includes an impressive battery of other nutrients: vitamin E, iron, selenium, omega-3, vitamin B6 and B9, fibre – to name but a few. This is why our mothers did their very best to feed us wheatgerm as children!

If you're gluten-intolerant, you'll need to avoid wheatgerm. And, as with everything, moderation is key.

Spermidine: we say

- Be sure to include some of the spermidine-rich ingredients listed above in your meals; however, if you're following a diverse plant-based diet, you're probably already getting plenty.
- We add the odd dessertspoonful of wheatgerm to our breakfast bowls.
- We often replace a tablespoon of flour with wheatgerm when baking.
- Always store wheatgerm in the fridge and eat it before its use-by date.
- If you don't like wheatgerm, try soya beans. Research suggests that, after wheatgerm, soya beans may have the highest levels of spermidine.[49]

Spice up your life

Herbs and spices have some of the highest concentrations of antioxidants on the planet. When we discovered just how rich in antioxidants and phytonutrients they were, we began adding them to anything and everything. But we didn't restrict ourselves to those routinely sold in plastic bags. Instead we planted many of the less-ubiquitous herbs and used them liberally in salads and stews. We also sought out unfamiliar spices and spice mixes, and used them as imaginatively as we could. Adding more herbs and spices to your daily cooking is one of the easiest (and most delicious) ways of helping your body and brain age well.

The free-radical theory of ageing speculates that many degenerative diseases result from the process of oxidation.[50] According to this theory, consuming antioxidants helps our bodies to age better. Many studies have suggested that increasing our intake of antioxidants could benefit our health, including a Swedish study of 30,000 women, which found that those with the most antioxidant-rich diets had the lowest risk of strokes, heart attacks and cataracts.[51]

The good news is that merely adding a pinch of the right spice or herb can hugely increase the antioxidant value of a meal. Half a teaspoon of cinnamon increases the antioxidant power of a bowl of porridge by 500 per cent. Add a pinch of cloves for a dazzling additional boost. Meanwhile, a single teaspoon of dried oregano can increase the antioxidant value of a plate of pasta by 400 per cent. Make that marjoram, and the value leaps still higher.[52]

It's hardly surprising, then, that so many herbs and spices are currently in some form of clinical trial. But it's not only the antioxidant value of herbs and spices that we appreciate. Both often contain anti-inflammatory compounds, and may also increase the diversity of our microbiome. Indeed, one spice appears to play such a profound anti-inflammatory role in the gut that we've devoted an entire section to it: turmeric.

Doctor Michael Greger has pored over the evidence for herbs and spices and found it suitably robust. His favourites are cloves, ginger, rosemary and turmeric (all four are anti-inflammatory and the subject of several clinical trials). He also rates allspice, basil, bay leaves, cardamom, cayenne, coriander, cumin, fenugreek, nutmeg, mustard, vanilla, saffron, paprika, lemongrass, lemon balm, marjoram, oregano, dill, parsley, peppermint (the most antioxidant-rich common herb of all), sage and thyme.[53]

Recent research suggests that a compound found in parsley and thyme (apigenin) helps brain function,[54] while other studies have found cinnamon to reduce cholesterol in diabetics.[55] We expect to see many more studies into the therapeutic power of herbs and spices. For now, though, we try to include at least one herb or spice in every savoury dish we cook.

- We like spice mixes for their ease and convenience and because, although a little more costly, they save wastage. Our favourites include za'atar, harissa, bharat and berbere.
- We plant mint, sage, parsley, thyme, basil and rosemary either in pots or in the garden.
- We also grow less common herbs such as lemon balm and sorrel, which we chop generously into salads and grain bowls.
- No garden? Herbs love a sunny windowsill.

- With strongly flavoured herbs such as rosemary and sage, we've learnt to use greater quantities than previously. Paired wisely, their flavours enhance rather than smother the flavours of other ingredients.
- Enjoy herb teas: ginger and peppermint – made with fresh mint leaves or a slice of fresh ginger – are two of our favourites.
- Keep a store of your favourite dried herbs (they have much higher levels of antioxidants, although we prefer fresh for flavour) beside the cooker so that it's easy to throw in a pinch as you go.
- Market stalls and ethnic food shops often sell large fresh bunches of herbs at a fraction of the price of the poly-thene-bagged herbs sold in supermarkets.
- Spices keep much longer if stored in the fridge.
- Sweet dishes can be herbed and spiced in exactly the same way. We like vanilla and cloves with stewed apples and plums, chopped mint, basil or lemon balm on ber-ries, cinnamon on sliced oranges, cloves and nutmeg with chocolate, and crystallised ginger with almost anything.·

Turmeric

Is turmeric the ultimate wonder-spice? A natural anti-inflammatory, it's been linked to a reduced risk of Alzheimer's, cancer and liver disease. It's also antiseptic, antibacterial and packed with antiox-idants. In India, where the spice is heavily consumed, fewer than one in 100 over-sixty-fives has Alzheimer's, whereas in the UK the figure is one in 14. Is it the turmeric?

Curcumin, the active ingredient that makes up around 3 per cent of turmeric, appears to counteract the low-grade, chronic inflammation that increases in our bodies as we age and contributes to many age-related diseases[56] – the so-called 'inflamm-ageing' discussed on page 28.

Research points to more benefits of curcumin in capsule form: in Austria it was shown to delay the liver damage that can lead to cirrhosis; at the University of Texas rodent studies suggested that curcumin might inhibit the growth of melanoma. Studies at the University of South Dakota found that pre-treatment with curcumin made cancer cells more vulnerable to chemo and radiotherapy.

It might also improve our brain function. A study at the UCLA Longevity Center found that older people with mild memory loss consuming 90mg of curcumin twice daily for 18 months had significant improvements in memory and attention span. Brain scans showed significantly less plaque and tangle accumulation (precursors to Alzheimer's disease) than in those taking placebos. As an added bonus, those taking curcumin also had mild improvements in mood.

That's not all. Curcumin supplementation has been shown to:

- Reduce pain, inflammation and stiffness in arthritis sufferers.
- Be as effective as Ibuprofen in reducing the pain of knee osteoarthritis.[57]
- Improve liver function.[58]
- Possibly have protective benefits against the risk of cancer.[59]
- Help irritable bowel syndrome and gut issues.[60]

Turmeric: we say

- Black pepper seems to increase absorption rates of curcumin, so we always try to combine it with turmeric.
- Keep turmeric close at hand – we keep a small tub on the kitchen counter so that it doesn't get forgotten.
- Add a teaspoonful to soups and stews (along with some black pepper) as well as curries and dhals.
- Think creatively: add a little to home-made hummus, or a hot milk drink to make a delicious latte.
- Make our turmeric sunrise tonic: a cup of warm water with 1 tablespoon apple cider vinegar, 1 teaspoon turmeric, ½ teaspoon black pepper, ½ teaspoon ginger pulp. Add honey to taste, stir well and enjoy as your first drink of the day.
- Don't go mad – turmeric is still being investigated, and all the experts we spoke to were very wary of any so-called superfoods. If you don't like it, don't worry.

Eat nuts

We're nuts about nuts. It's a cliché, but it's true. They deliver extraordinary Age-Well benefits and taste fantastic, so what's not to love? (Unless you're allergic, of course.) Their positive impact on health is far ranging: the risk of a number of age-related diseases and conditions reduces when we eat nuts regularly, so we introduced them early on in our Age-Well Project.

We added a daily handful of raw nuts to our diets after a review of 29 studies from around the world concluded that,

'Higher nut intake is associated with reduced risk of cardiovascular disease, total cancer and all-cause mortality, and
mortality from respiratory disease, diabetes, and infection.'
The report showed that a large handful (about 28g) of nuts per
day was enough to reduce the risk of coronary heart disease by
almost one-third and the risk of all cancers by 15 per cent. Nut
consumption also slashed respiratory disease risk in half, and
reduced type-2 diabetes risk by 40 per cent.[61]

Other studies have confirmed the positive impact of eating
nuts on heart health: data gathered from over 210,000 people
over 30 years revealed a 14 per cent lower risk of cardiovascular
disease and a 20 per cent lower risk of coronary heart disease for
those eating nuts five times a week. But eating nuts two to four
times a week was also beneficial. The lead researcher explained:
'Nuts can be beneficial for health because they're high in unsaturated fatty acids, dietary fibre, minerals, vitamins, and other
bioactive compounds. And there's some evidence that nuts can
improve blood lipids, attenuate inflammation, benefit endothelial
function and decrease insulin resistance.'[62]

The positive impact of nuts on 'bad' cholesterol is echoed in
other reports. A study investigating the effects of nuts (pistachio
nuts, pine nuts, pecan nuts, macadamia nuts, hazelnuts, Brazil
nuts, almonds and, particularly, walnuts) on cholesterol, blood
pressure and inflammation found that eating nuts lowers LDL
(aka 'bad') cholesterol, triglycerides and ApoB (which helps
deliver fat to cells and is indicated in the build-up of plaques in
the arteries, leading to atherosclerosis).[63]

Walnuts seem to be the star of the nut world. A study from
Tufts University in the US found that eating walnuts made lab
rats 'younger and smarter', leading researchers to conclude
that eating seven to nine walnuts daily could delay the onset of

Alzheimer's and dementia. They believe walnuts might curb oxidative damage to brain cells, fight inflammation and stimulate the birth of new neurons.

Further research has focused on the effect of nuts on the brain. A 2017 study used an electroencephalogram (EEG) to examine the brain waves of regular nut eaters. Nuts are rich in flavonoids, which have been found to boost the hippocampus (the part of the brain responsible for learning and memory) by encouraging the growth of new neurons and increasing blood flow. The nut eaters showed an increase in delta and gamma waves in the brain, believed to improve the REM sleep where memories are laid down.[64]

Nuts: we say

- Brazil nuts are high in selenium, which supports healthy thyroid function and the immune system: we keep a tub close at hand to snack on. Three or four provide all the selenium we need each day.
- Pistachio nuts, quite apart from looking beautiful, are rich in vitamin B_6, which keeps hormones balanced. They also contain lutein: an antioxidant that plays an important role in protecting our eyes. Sprinkle them, chopped, over grain salads and porridge.
- Walnuts contain high levels of omega-3 for brain and skin health. Try toasting them and blending them with kale, olive oil and a little hard cheese to make a pesto.
- Almonds are rich in calcium, helping prevent osteoporosis – a major concern for ageing women.

- Experiment with nut butters: walnut, crunchy cashew, smooth almond – they're all delicious. Spread on toast, use to top porridge or blend into sauces and dips.

What about the calories?

Unless you're eating jarfuls of nuts, don't fret about the calories. A handful of nuts can contain up to 200 calories, but studies show that adding nuts to your diet won't lead to weight gain if you're replacing less healthy snacks.[65]

Olive oil

We think of olive oil as liquid gold, such is its potency. Indeed, some of the protective benefits of the much-lauded Mediterranean diet may come from this one ingredient.

Olive oil differs from seed oils because it's pressed from the whole fruit rather than extracted from a seed (often using chemical solvents). The first pressing, known as extra virgin olive oil, is the richest in nutrients. The olives can be pressed many more times, but later pressings are less nutritious. The oil used in research trials, and referred to in this chapter, is extra virgin olive oil.

During our Age-Well Project we eliminated most seed oils, fell in and out of love with coconut oil, but always remained faithful to olive oil. Why? It seems that olive oil provides numerous health benefits, with improved heart health topping the list. A four-and-a-half-year clinical trial involving 7,000 older adults at risk of heart disease found that those eating an olive-oil rich Mediterranean diet had 30 per cent fewer instances of heart attacks, strokes, memory loss and breast cancer, as well as improved lipid and cholesterol levels and blood pressure.[66]

The antioxidant properties of olive oil appear to protect our hearts and blood vessels by fighting the oxidative stress that damages the heart and hardens the arteries.[67] Oleic acid, a monounsaturated fat and the main component of olive oil, raises 'good' (HDL) cholesterol and lowers 'bad' (LDL). The polyphenols found in olive oil help to protect cholesterol in our blood from oxidation. The combination of oleic acid and polyphenols is also thought to reduce blood pressure. In a small study, high-blood-pressure sufferers fed olive oil saw their levels reduce dramatically, with some able to come off medication altogether.[68]

Olive oil can also play a role in:

Cancer It might lower the rate of some cancers by decreasing oxidative stress in our cells and protecting DNA from oxidative damage. It might also slow the progression of breast cancer.[69]

Brain health A French study found that older people using olive oil had better visual memory and verbal fluency than those who used none.[70]

Metabolic syndrome and diabetes The polyphenols in olive oil might aid these conditions by decreasing body weight, blood pressure and blood glucose.[71]

Osteoporosis Evidence suggests that olive oil polyphenols might prevent the loss of bone mass.[72]

The gut Olive oil might help to balance gut bacteria and prevent the overgrowth of bad bacteria. Over 80 per cent of olive oil's fatty acids make it to the gut, where they feed our microbiome.

Olive oil: we say

- Don't fall for 'pure' olive oil or other terms indicating the oil is a mix of extra virgin and other types. Use extra virgin olive oil.
- Look for 'cold pressed' or 'first pressing' in preference.
- Buy extra virgin olive oil in dark glass bottles. The tinted glass protects the active compounds in the oil and prevents it going rancid.
- No one consumes olive oil on its own. Use it to cook, or dress, polyphenol-rich multi-coloured vegetables. It might be the combination and interaction of nutrients that make them so beneficial as we age.
- A drizzle of good-quality olive oil over a dish of vegetables or meat/fish makes a huge difference to the taste and the amount of nutrients we absorb.
- Switching from vegetable oils to olive oil has been shown to improve cholesterol levels: we use very few vegetable and seed oils now, and rarely for cooking.

Coconut oil

Just why is coconut oil so trendy? It became the ultimate 'superfood' after research published in 2009 linked it to weight loss and higher levels of HDL 'good' cholesterol.[73] Suddenly it was everywhere. But it's a divisive subject.

In 2017 the American Heart Association published a 'presidential advisory'[74] on the subject, advising against the use of coconut oil. The Association suggested that the saturated fat in coconut oil could raise 'bad' (LDL) cholesterol. Eighty-two per cent of the fat in coconut oil is saturated, as opposed to 63 per cent in butter and 50 per cent in beef fat. And, to add fuel to the coconut oil fire, Professor Karin Michels, an epidemiologist at Harvard's School of Public Health, described it as 'pure poison'. Like the AHA, she took issue with the high level of saturated fat. Many other health experts have argued against this, pointing out that the AHA used outdated research to back their findings and only looked at total fat intake, not coconut oil specifically.

Coconut oil might have a positive role to play in brain health, however. Our brains use glucose as fuel. But if glucose supplies run low, the brain can function on an alternative fuel source – ketones – which are produced in the liver when carbohydrate stores are low. Ketones are also found in MCT (medium-chain triglyceride) oil, usually derived from coconuts. As we age, the brain becomes less efficient at using glucose. This is particularly true of the Alzheimer's brain, which can't use glucose efficiently so is, effectively, starving. Studies indicate that supplementing the diet of dementia patients with MCT oil, or putting them on a high-fat, low-carb ketogenic diet,[75] has a beneficial effect on brain energy metabolism.[76]

Hundreds of other reports on the power of coconut oil have been published, although the research often takes the form of rodent, rather than human studies. But coconut oil has been credited with several benefits:

- Improving antioxidant levels[77] (thereby slowing the ageing process), and reducing inflammation in arthritic rats.
- Working as a natural antibiotic by disrupting the lipid coating on bacteria. Lauric acid in coconut oil can create a hostile environment for viruses and bacteria in the body[78] – meaning fewer bugs and colds.
- Preventing bone loss in post-menopausal rats.[79]
- And – the icing on the mid-life-woman's cake – coconut oil might have a positive effect on the menopause itself by aiding oestrogen levels.

The conversation about coconut oil isn't over yet. Yes, saturated fat levels are very high. But a report in 2018[80] suggested that when compared to butter, coconut oil consumption led to lower LDL ('bad') and higher HDL ('good') cholesterol, in contrast to the 2017 study noted above. Experts believe more research is needed.[81] Meanwhile, we'll continue using it from time to time.

Coconut oil: we say

- Buy organic raw virgin coconut oil – not the processed variety, which is made from the copra (heated dried coconut) and not the fresh coconut flesh and is impure and less nutritious.
- If you're trying coconut oil for the first time, use a small amount. It can cause upset stomachs and diarrhoea if you start with too much.
- We use it for frying pancakes. It imparts a lovely sweet taste.

- It makes a good base for curries: fry onions, garlic and spices in coconut oil before adding the other ingredients.
- It's solid at room temperature, so it makes a useful addition to raw cookies or energy balls, helping to hold them together.
- If you're concerned about high cholesterol, talk to your doctor about using coconut oil.
- Coconut oil also makes a great, chemical-free skin moisturiser and make-up remover.

Red meat

We're often asked if we've renounced red meat. We haven't. For us, it's about eating better quality meat, in moderation and alongside plenty of vegetables.

After years of reading research we've come to the conclusion that a diet packed with vegetables, fruit, pulses, fish and whole grains is best for our long-term health. But that doesn't preclude the occasional piece of meat. In the journal *Current Developments in Nutrition*, a group of academics suggested that eating red meat, or not, was irrelevant to a good diet. What increased the risk of heart disease and diabetes was whether or not the red meat was lean and unprocessed, and what *else* was in the diet. Like us, the researchers concluded that a nutrient-rich diet was not undone by the occasional serving of good-quality red meat.[82] When we interviewed JoAnn Manson, Professor of Women's Health at Harvard Medical School, she concurred. 'A small amount of red meat – don't eat it daily – can fit into a healthy diet. You don't have to be vegetarian or vegan. It comes down to whole foods as opposed to processed ones, if you're having lots of fruit, vegetables, whole grains, nuts, legumes, fish, and other whole foods, a little red meat is OK.'

Red meat is high in vitamins B_{12}, B_3, and B_6, and rich in easily absorbed forms of iron, zinc, selenium, sodium, phosphorus and potassium: all nutrients critical to our diet, so why *shouldn't* we eat it?

Red meat was demonised until recently because of its saturated fat content, which doctors thought caused high blood pressure, soaring cholesterol and, ultimately, heart attacks. New research has revealed a different picture. A review of randomised controlled trials found that consumption of small amounts of red meat (around 35g a day) had no effect on blood pressure or cholesterol levels.[83] However, the World Health Organization classifies red meat as Group 2A, 'probably carcinogenic to humans'.[84] The Organization states, 'The strongest, but still limited, evidence for an association with eating red meat is for colorectal cancer.' More than 2.2 million new cases of colorectal (bowel) cancer are expected worldwide by 2030. Numerous studies and reviews have linked higher intake of red and processed meat to a higher risk of colorectal cancer.[85]

Cancer isn't the only health issue linked to red meat. Research has found that increased consumption of red and processed meat led to an increased risk for diabetes[86] and non-alcoholic fatty liver disease.[87]

Global meat consumption has soared in recent decades, leading to ethical concerns about its production and environmental impact. Research from Oxford University found that meat and dairy production provide just 18 per cent of calories and 37 per cent of protein consumed worldwide, but use over 80 per cent of farmland and produce more than half of agriculture's greenhouse gas emissions.[88] Many of the experts we spoke to while writing this book eat little or no red meat. They cited both health reasons and concerns about the environmental impact of raising livestock.

Red meat: we say

- If you want to eat red meat as part of a healthy diet, then do. But think about how much, how often, how best to cook it and its provenance.
- Your butcher should know the provenance and feeding patterns of his/her meat. Don't be afraid to ask. Supermarket butchers are often as knowledgeable as specialist butchers.
- Cooking methods make a huge difference. Meat that's been grilled or fried is likely to contain advanced glycation end-products (AGEs), which have been linked to cancer and diabetes.
- Braise, stew or marinate your meat: one study found that people fed marinated red meat had fewer biomarkers for colon cancer.[89]
- These cooking methods work well with cheaper cuts of meat, making them more economical too.
- The NHS Bowel Cancer Screening Programme offers screening to all men and women over 55. When offered a test – take it.

Berries (and cherries)

We've eaten plenty of blueberries since starting our Age-Well project. And blackberries. And blackcurrants. And raspberries. And strawberries. Oh, and cherries, too. We're not jumping on the 'superfood' bandwagon for the sake of it: a stack of research reveals the health benefits of these delicious fruits.

As with highly coloured vegetables, berries and cherries contain powerful flavonoids. Red, blue and purple fruits are rich in anthocyanins (literally 'blue plants'), antioxidants that fight damage to the body from free radicals – the unstable atoms that harm cells, causing ageing and disease.

The most compelling research points to the impact of berries on cognitive decline and brain ageing. Eating more berries seems to help the brain's neurons communicate with each other, reducing age-related decline.[90] Research data from a study of more than 120,000 women found that those who ate more blueberries and strawberries had a slower rate of cognitive decline. The researchers observed that women who ate more berries delayed cognitive ageing by up to two and a half years.[91] They also noted that eating more berries is, as they put it, 'a fairly simple dietary modification' which could have a huge impact on brain health as we age.

A very small study of people with mild cognitive decline found that consuming wild blueberry juice for 12 weeks led to improved memory and reduced depressive symptoms.[92] A more detailed study, using mice, found that 14 weeks of supplementation with polyphenol-rich grape and blueberry extract prevented age-related learning and memory problems.[93]

Fresh berries also have an impact on heart health: they can significantly reduce the build-up of LDL (the so-called 'bad' cholesterol).

Researchers looked at data from over 1,200 people and found that people who regularly ate berries had lower levels of LDL, which contributes to heart disease, stroke and atherosclerosis.[94]

There's an entire project at the University of East Anglia (UEA) dedicated to investigating the health benefits of blueberries.[95] Their research found that women who ate three or more portions of blueberries and strawberries each week had fewer heart attacks.[96] The researchers suggested that anthocyanins might help to dilate blood vessels and counter plaque build-up in the arteries. The same team also found that eating berries could help reduce high blood pressure.

Some of the most interesting research to come out of the UEA links high levels of anthocyanins to a reduced risk of type-2 diabetes.[97] Eating more berries was linked to lower insulin resistance and better blood glucose regulation. The researchers said, 'We found that those who consumed plenty of anthocyanins and flavones had lower insulin resistance. High insulin resistance is associated with type-2 diabetes, so people who eat foods rich in these compounds – such as berries, herbs, red grapes, wine – are less likely to develop the disease.'

The anthocyanins from berries have also shown promise in cancer treatment. They increase the function of an enzyme called sirtuin 6. Sirtuins are naturally occurring enzymes in our bodies that regulate the expression of genes that control cell function. Sirtuins change as we age, making us more likely to develop diseases such as cancer. But the anthocyanins in berries have been shown to increase sirtuin 6 activity, which in turn might reduce cancer cell growth.[98] This doesn't mean that eating a handful of berries will reduce tumour growth, but it's an avenue for scientists to explore as they continue uncovering the power of these wonder-fruits.

Berries: we say

- Eat a few berries every day.
- A freezer is your best friend: frozen blueberries and raspberries are so much cheaper than fresh. A handful – straight from the freezer – works perfectly in porridge, overnight oats and smoothies.
- Forage: we pick hedgerow blackberries in late summer/ early autumn for our freezers. This is free, wild, food packed with Age-Well nutrients – what could be better? Although we avoid berries growing beside busy roads.
- Exotic 'superfood' fruit such as goji berries and acai are also full of polyphenols and anthocyanins. Experiment with them if you like, but we prefer seasonal, local produce.
- Cherries are one of the few natural sources of melatonin – meaning that they'll also help you to sleep better.
- Blackcurrant bushes are exceptionally easy to grow and contain more antioxidants, vitamins and minerals than any other berry. Plant the newer varieties, which are as fat and sweet as blueberries (we like 'Big Ben'). Forget topping and tailing, and serve as they are.
- Berries and cherries aren't just for desserts and breakfasts – add them to salads or use in a sauce for meat or poultry.

Miraculous mushrooms

Mushrooms are the perfect Age-Well food: rich in essential amino acids, vitamins (B_1, B_2, B_{12}, C, D and E) and trace minerals such as zinc and selenium. The vitamin D content is particularly important, as mushrooms are the only plant-based source of this much-needed nutrient. They're a source of fibre, particularly the soluble fibre beta glucan, which can lower blood cholesterol levels and boost immunity. Mushrooms contain choline, which helps with sleep, muscle movement, learning and memory. Choline also assists in maintaining the structure of cellular membranes, transmitting nerve impulses, supporting fat absorption and reducing chronic inflammation.

Mushrooms contain high amounts of two antioxidants, ergothioneine and glutathione, both critical for ageing well. When we digest food, free radicals can appear as a by-product. Their accumulation in the body has been associated with many ageing diseases including cancer, heart disease and Alzheimer's. Research shows that our bodies use the antioxidants in mushrooms to mop up these free radicals.[99] Porcini mushrooms are a particularly rich source of antioxidants. Researchers suggest that the lower incidence of neurodegenerative diseases in Mediterranean countries might be linked to the love of mushrooms in Southern Europe.

There's a huge variety of mushrooms, all with slightly different health benefits. Shiitake are considered good immune boosters, whereas maitake have been shown to reduce hypertension and inflammation.[100] But if you can't find, or afford, the more exotic mushrooms, fear not. The humble white button mushroom has as much, and in some cases, more, antioxidant properties than its more glamorous cousins. A team of French researchers found that the white button mushroom was as good at cleaning up free radicals as other mushrooms. A Chinese study found that eating mushrooms, particularly white button mushrooms, was associated with a lower risk of ovarian cancer in women over 50.[101] And elderly rats fed an extract of white button mushrooms showed improvements in balance and working memory.[102]

White button mushrooms have also been found to modify gut microbiota in mice.[103] The mushrooms act as powerful prebiotics, boosting beneficial bacteria, which leads to improved blood sugar control. The researchers believe that mushrooms ferment in the gut, triggering microbiotic growth, which, in turn, leads to the expression of genes involved in the production of glucose. Managing glucose is, of course, critical for diabetes treatment and other metabolic diseases.

Mushrooms: we say

- The vitamin D content of mushrooms can be increased by leaving them in the sun (a sunny windowsill is perfect) for an hour or two.
- Unless you know what you're doing, don't forage for wild mushrooms without an expert to guide you.
- The meaty texture of mushrooms makes them the perfect replacement for animal products in many dishes.
- Large portobello mushrooms are delicious stuffed with chopped nuts, cheese and herbs, then baked.
- Use a wide variety of mushrooms; all have different health benefits.

- Research suggests that the nutritional value of mushrooms is better preserved when grilled or microwaved, as opposed to deep-frying.
- Dried porcini mushrooms are easy to find. Soak 20g in warm water for 30 minutes, then squeeze dry, finely chop and add to a risotto or stew. Don't waste the soaking liquid: strain and add to your cooking, leaving the sediment behind.

CHAPTER 6

What to Drink

If you are what you eat, you're also what you drink. Simple changes to what – and how – we consume liquids can make a dramatic difference when it comes to ageing well. In this chapter we reveal how we've transformed our relationship with alcohol, the best ways of imbibing tea and coffee and how to drink more water.

Rethink alcohol

Several studies now link *moderate* (and this is the single most important word on this page) drinking with reduced overall mortality. A small regular drink, it appears, might lower our risk of cardiovascular disease, hypertension, diabetes, cognitive impairment/dementia and certain cancers, including colon, basal cell, ovarian and prostate.[1] Scientists don't know what it is in alcohol that seems to protect us. Is it the ethanol? Or is it the phytonutrients from the grapes and hops? Or is it something else altogether? So far, the evidence points to the phytonutrients, as spirits don't appear to have the same beneficial effects – in fact, there's no evidence they have any benefit whatsoever.

Enjoy a guilt-free glass of beer

Although red wine – with its greater count of phytonutrients[2] – remains the preferred tipple of most longevity experts, there's no need to write off beer just yet. Indeed beer contains, measure for measure, fewer calories, and less sugar and alcohol than wine. Most compellingly of all, moderate beer drinkers, like their fellow red-wine imbibers, have a lower risk of cardiovascular and neurodegenerative disease.[3]

An Italian study of 200,000 people found that moderate beer drinkers had a 31 per cent lower risk of heart attacks, strokes and heart disease.[4] They were also found to have a lower risk of developing kidney stones.[5]

Beer might have particular benefits for mid-life women, too. A Spanish study declared its potent blend of antioxidants, vitamins, nutrients, fibre and phytoestrogens to be 'highly beneficial in the prevention of pathologies arising from the decline in oestrogens' at menopause, as well as possibly reducing the risk of osteoporosis.[6] That's because beer is a good source of dietary silicon, vital for bones.[7] A study of 2,700 people found that those who consumed more silicon had higher bone density. It's not just our bones that need silicon. Our skin, nails and tendons all require collagen, which in turn requires silicon. A half-pint of beer is thought to have around 8mg of silicon, along with vitamins B_2, B_6, B_9 and B_{12}.[8]

Finally, beer contains a flavonoid called xanthohumol, which is found only in hops. A study of mice found that a diet of xanthohumol improved their spatial memory and cognitive flexibility.[9] OK, so you'd need to drink 2,000 litres of beer to get the same effect as a mouse in that study – but research like this reminds us that even beer might contain a little bit of goodness.

On the other hand, it's possible that moderate beer drinkers are protected by something else altogether. Could it be the social engagement that comes from enjoying an occasional social beer? Or is it the walk to and from the pub?

We don't know. But if you fancy a beer, have one. Perhaps just half a pint. And perhaps not every day. A recent study linked drinking more than five pints of beer a week to a lower life expectancy.[10]

In our experience, low and alcohol-free beers often taste as good as the real deal. Indeed we've participated in blind tastings where seasoned beer drinkers were unable to spot the difference. We often enjoy an alcohol-free beer, which provides the best of all possible worlds.

- For maximum bone-building silicon, choose beer based on barley rather than wheat.
- Paler/lighter ales are subject to less heat during the malting process, so they contain more silicon and other phytonutrients. In one study, India Pale Ale (IPA) came tops in terms of silicon content, whereas non-alcoholic and wheat beers and light lagers had the least.[11]
- Unsure what moderate is? Guidelines vary, and so does the alcohol content of different beers. In the UK the recommendation is for no more than six pints of beer a week, but a study in the *Lancet* recommends no more than five at 4 per cent ABV (alcohol by volume, or the alcohol percentage). You can find guidelines at www.drinkaware.co.uk.

- Avoid any confusion and switch to low- or no-alcohol beers to enjoy the nutritional benefits without the alcohol (although the silicon content will be less).

Drink wine – but make it red, and drink with consciousness

Drinking becomes more risky as we age. We're less able to metabolise alcohol (because of our slower rates of elimination and lower volumes of total body water) and some of the medical conditions that come with growing older (high blood pressure, for example) can be exacerbated by alcohol. Should we drink at all? And if so, what should we drink?

The World Health Organization's International Agency for Research on Cancer classifies alcohol as a Group 1 carcinogen, putting it in the same league table as asbestos and tobacco. Numerous studies have linked alcohol consumption to seven forms of cancer: liver, colon, rectum, larynx, oropharynx, oesophagus and breast. Until recently, scientists weren't sure why this was so, but a new study suggests that acetaldehyde, the chemical produced when our bodies break down alcohol, damages DNA within our blood stem cells, permanently altering DNA sequences and making our cells more vulnerable to cancer.[12]

It's not only the risk of cancer that rises with alcohol consumption, however. Many studies have linked heavy drinking (more than 14 units, or seven medium glasses a week) with Alzheimer's and dementia. It's now thought that 10 per cent of dementia cases might be alcohol-related. A Finnish study found middle-aged binge-drinkers (defined as a bottle of wine in an evening, twice a month or more) were three times more likely to develop dementia, 25 years later.[13]

Despite this, there's a strong body of evidence to suggest that alcohol in moderation has some general longevity benefits. Residents of the Blue Zones (the areas of the world with the greatest number of centenarians) typically drink moderate but regular quantities of alcohol – robust local wines in Ikaria and Sardinia, for example. In the 90+ study of SuperAgers, alcohol is consumed regularly, prompting researcher Professor Claudia Kawas to say that she had no explanation for it but that she firmly believes modest drinking 'improves longevity.'[14]

Researchers at the William Harvey Research Institute found that the high levels of procyanidins in red wine improved the function of the linings of blood vessels,[15] thus reducing the risk of heart disease, strokes, diabetes, dementia and possibly some cancers. A long-term study of data from 19 nations found a statistically significant lower risk of dementia among regular, moderate red wine drinkers in 14 countries,[16] confirmed in a recent meta-analysis, which concluded that teetotallers and heavy drinkers (more than 14 units – seven medium glasses – of wine a week) had a greater risk of dementia than those drinking between one and 14 units.[17]

Another study found that moderate red wine drinking boosted levels of omega-3s in the red blood cells[18] while a study from Johns Hopkins University suggested that red wine could shield the brain from stroke damage.[19] Another report suggested that red wine could stop the proliferation of lung cancer cells and boost lung function.[20]

A study published in the *Journal of the American College of Cardiology* found that moderate drinking (between 3 and 14 drinks per week for men, and 7 or fewer for women) might have protective effects against cardiovascular disease. The researchers reported that 'A delicate balance exists between the beneficial and detrimental effects of alcohol consumption. A J-shaped relationship exists between alcohol consumption and mortality, and drinkers should drink with consciousness.'

Scientists still don't understand exactly how red wine in moderation helps us. Many have suggested it's a polyphenol called resveratrol that is found in wine. We've weighed up the evidence (which is by no means conclusive) and until there's a better understanding of how wine helps or harms, we're determined to enjoy the odd glass.

Wine: we say

- Drink traditionally produced (where the fermentation period is a month rather than a week) red wines with a high procyanidin content, like Madiran from Gascony or wines from the Nuoro area of Sardinia. Cabernet Sauvignon and Nebbiolo grapes appear to make the wine with the highest levels of procyanidins
- Red wine is not just for winter – drink it lightly chilled in summer.
- Grapes are heavily sprayed. Choose organic or biodynamic if you can.
- Have at least two alcohol-free days every week.
- Stick to the guidelines: experts suggest a single 150–175ml glass a day for women and two for men (although that falls to one for men over the age of 65).
- Savour rather than guzzle (that is, drink with consciousness).
- Never mix alcohol and over-the-counter or prescription drugs.

- If you've a family predisposition to cancer, weigh up the evidence very carefully and consider drastically reducing your wine consumption until research consistently suggests otherwise.
- Worried about the odd report stating that 'There's no safe level of alcohol'? Don't be. There's no safe level of driving, flying in an aeroplane or crossing the road either.

Green tea

If there's a panacea for the world's ailments, it's green tea. Or so it seems. Research has credited this simple drink with reducing the risk of, or improving outcomes for, cognitive decline, cancer, diabetes, obesity, heart disease and arthritis. Green tea is also packed with antioxidants, reducing free-radical damage to our bodies. A Japanese study followed 40,000 40- to 79-year-olds for 11 years and found that green tea drinkers had a substantially lower risk of death from *all* causes (yes – all!).[21]

The active compound in green tea is EGCG (epigallocatechin-3-gallate), which researchers have linked to a wide variety of possible health benefits. No one's suggesting a cup of green tea can prevent cancer, diabetes or heart disease. But green tea extract, EGCG, *could* be used to prevent or treat the following conditions:

Cognitive decline and type-2 diabetes Research published in China suggested that EGCG could alleviate the insulin resistance and cognitive impairment which result from a typical Western diet. The researchers put mice on a high-fat, high-sugar diet and gave half of them an EGCG solution. Those drinking the EGCG had a lower body weight after three months, and performed better in cognitive tests. Author Dr Xuebo Liu said. 'The ancient habit of drinking green tea may be a more acceptable alternative to medicine when it comes to combatting obesity, insulin resistance, and memory impairment.'[22]

Cancer tumours Research from Korea found that dosing cancerous mice with EGCG inhibited tumour growth and tumour cell proliferation.[23] Additionally, a team from the University of Strathclyde found a way to deliver EGCG directly to cancer tumours – which caused the tumours to shrink. In two different types of skin cancer, 40 per cent of tumours vanished.[24]

Alzheimer's disease It seems that EGCG reduces the accumulation of the toxic plaques of beta-amyloid in the brain associated with Alzheimer's. Researchers at McMaster University in Canada discovered that EGCG prevents tiny molecules of beta-amyloid clumping together, essentially by remodelling them.[25]

Heart disease and stroke Consumption of green tea has been linked to improved functioning of the cells lining the arteries, making them more supple and helping blood to flow more easily.[26]

Arthritis A study found that EGCG inhibited the production of those molecules in the immune system that contribute to inflammation in connective tissue and joint damage.[27]

Green tea: we say

- If you don't like the taste, add a squeeze of lemon –
  the vitamin C gives staying power to the antioxidants
  in the tea.
- Try iced green tea in summer. Brew it, let it cool, then add
  ice. It's delicious.
- Buy the best-quality loose-leaf green tea you can afford,
  and prepare it carefully.
- Don't use boiling water – take the kettle off the boil as
  soon as bubbles start to form on the surface of the water,
  or let it cool to 70–80°C.
- Use around 1 teaspoon of tea per cup.
- Don't leave the tea steeping for long, as this makes
  it bitter.
- But don't be afraid to re-use the tea by topping up the
  pot with hot water. The thrifty Chinese say the third cup
  is the best.

Wake up and smell the … beneficial coffee

The case for drinking coffee is mounting. The last few years have
seen multiple studies suggesting that coffee could:

- Lower the risk of death from heart failure or stroke.
- Reduce the chance of premature death in women
  with diabetes.
- Help stave off Parkinson's and Alzheimer's disease.

- Halve the risk of prostate cancer, while reducing the risk of several other cancers.[28]

Recently, a team of researchers from the University of Southampton examined all the data from more than 200 observational studies and clinical trials. They found that coffee consumption was linked to a decrease in the risk of cardiovascular disease, cancer, non-alcoholic fatty liver disease, cirrhosis and diabetes. More specifically, they found that three cups of coffee a day lowered the risk of coronary heart disease by 19 per cent; lowered the chances of dying from a stroke by 30 per cent; and lowered the risk of developing liver cirrhosis by 39 per cent.

Overall, coffee consumption correlated with a lower risk of mortality from *all* causes, leading the researchers to conclude that moderate coffee consumption – four cups a day or the equivalent of 400mg of caffeine – is 'more likely to benefit health than to harm'.[29] This echoes a 2017 Spanish study of 19,000 people that found participants who had at least four daily cups of coffee had a 65 per cent lower risk of dying from all causes, compared with those who said they never or rarely drank coffee.[30]

Do these benefits extend to people drinking more than four to five cups a day? An even newer report suggests that they do, finding those people drinking eight cups a day enjoyed the same protection, independent of whether they were fast or slow metabolisers of caffeine. In this study instant coffee was found to have slightly fewer benefits.[31]

We wouldn't go this far. In fact, we'd err on the side of caution and stick with the advice of The 90+ Study, [32] which found that the longest-living people enjoyed two to four cups a day.

Is it the caffeine or is it the antioxidants? Or perhaps the polyphenols? Researchers aren't sure. Coffee is rich in both antioxidants and polyphenols, and some scientists believe it's these that give coffee its protective powers. Other studies suggest it's the caffeine that counts and that caffeine may have anti-inflammatory properties. A recent study found that older people with low levels of inflammation – which drives most ageing diseases – all consumed caffeine.[33]

A study from the Krembil Brain Institute now claims to have identified the magic ingredient (possibly): phenylindanes, a group of compounds made during the roasting process that appears to inhibit the clumping of beta-amyloid and tau commonly found in the brains of those with Parkinson's and Alzheimer's diseases. This study also found dark-roasted coffee (caffeinated or decaff) to have higher quantities of phenylindanes.[34]

Coffee: we say

- Enjoy guilt-free caffeinated coffee unless you're a child/ teen, pregnant or lactating (where the dangers of caffeine might outweigh the benefits).
- Avoid caffeine after 4pm. It can take up to seven hours to be metabolised.
- Choose dark roasted over light roasted.
- Take your coffee unsweetened and avoid processed flavoured syrups.
- Consider cutting the milk – one study showed the antioxidant value of coffee was 'significantly reduced' when milk was added.[35]
- Go organic if you can – coffee is heavily sprayed with pesticides.

Water – drink up!

We all know how vital water is to good health. But staying hydrated becomes increasingly important as we age, not least because our sense of thirst diminishes as we get older. Age interferes with the systems that control thirst, so we're less aware of the need to drink.[36] The hypothalamus (the part of the brain that monitors the blood's concentration of sodium and toxins) sends out a signal telling us to drink. But, as we age, that system becomes less sensitive.

An Australian study gave salty water to two groups of participants, an older group (aged 65–74) and a younger group (aged 21–30), to make them thirsty. Both groups were then allowed to drink as much plain water as they wanted. The older group only drank half as much water as the youngsters. Brain imaging of the older group showed that the area of the brain that predicts how much water is needed switched off before they'd drunk enough.[37]

The total water content of our bodies declines as we age. When we're born, we're about 70 per cent water; by the age of 60, that's decreased to around 52 per cent in men and 46 per cent in women, mainly due to decreased muscle mass. Our kidneys aren't able to conserve water as well as they could when we were younger, but they need more to detoxify our systems. Therefore, just as there's less water in the body, we require more.

Sleep deprivation is also linked to dehydration. Vasopressin, a hormone that controls the body's water balance, is released late in the sleep cycle.[38] If we wake too early, which is more likely as we age, the hormone doesn't fulfil its function and we become dehydrated (as well as tired).

As our water reserves become depleted, cognitive function

declines too. Research shows that cognition and concentration decrease severely with about a 2 per cent decline in body mass due to dehydration.[39] That can happen after exercise, or after working hard in the garden on a hot day. Add to that the cognitive decline which happens naturally with age, and the importance of water to our brains is clear. The good news is that all this can be resolved by . . . water: free and from nothing more complicated than a tap!

Water: we say

- Invest in a water filtration system, or at least a filter jug. There's nothing wrong with tap water, but the purer our drinking water, the better.
- How much to drink each day? NHS guidelines say 1.2 litres a day, US guidelines are higher, recommending almost 2 litres daily. But . . .
- . . . as thirst is not a reliable indicator of how much water we need over the age of 50, keep an eye on the colour of your urine. If it's any darker than straw, you're dehydrated.
- Finding plain water boring? Flavour it with fresh mint, lemon slices, cucumber strips or berries.
- Teas and infusions are hydrating. We like fresh mint, chamomile (especially before bed), liquorice, ginger and nettle.
- Keep a water bottle in your bag, by your bed, on your desk, in your car . . .
- We prefer stainless steel water bottles to plastic. Plastic degrades, leaching chemicals over time.

- Vegetables and fruit are high in water. Include lettuce, cucumber, celery and spinach – the vegetables with the highest water content – in your diet to help you stay hydrated.
- Some medication, including over-the-counter cold remedies, can be dehydrating. Increase your water intake and talk to your doctor if you're concerned.

CORNERSTONE TWO

Exercise

Every expert we interviewed for this book emphasised the importance of exercise. JoAnn Manson, Professor of Women's Health at Harvard Medical School, told us, 'The magic bullet for good health is staying physically active. It affects every other factor: blood pressure, insulin sensitivity, blood sugar, cholesterol levels, body weight and inflammation levels. Everything is improved by regular physical activity.'

Meir Stampfer, Professor of Medicine at Harvard Medical School, agrees: 'Taking exercise is the number one change people can make. If you're completely inactive it will change your life, so it's a big shift.'

In this section we explore why moving your body – every hour and every day – is vital for healthy longevity. Research shows that people who get less than 20 minutes of exercise a day have the highest risk of death, whereas those doing more than 60 minutes reduce their risk of death by 57 per cent.[1] Crucially, we're not talking here about an hour in the gym: bite-sized chunks of exercise spread across the day might be more effective. Nor

*does it need to be hardcore. A brisk stroll, carrying bags of shop-
ping, vacuuming or a game of ping-pong all count. We've tried
everything from fidgeting to ballroom dancing, from rowing to
yoga, from digging the garden to lifting weights. When it comes
to ageing better, anything goes.*

CHAPTER 7

How to Move

Want to live longer? Then get up and move – every 30 minutes. This is the advice of scientists who found that prolonged sitting dramatically increases our risk of premature death. As people with desk jobs, this was a message we couldn't afford to ignore.

This section includes several suggestions for increasing your fitness and avoiding being too sedentary. As before, we suggest that you look through our 'We say' boxes and select the type of exercise that might suit you. If you're unused to exercise, start slowly and gently. You're aiming for progression not perfection: any exercise is better than none. For an overview, see also our brief explanation of this section in the Introduction.

Sitting – an unnatural way of living

The average adult now spends 9–12 hours a day sitting. And it's killing us – even when we bookend our sedentary days with bursts of frenzied exercise. According to the World Health Organization, sedentary behaviour now ranks among the ten leading causes of death.

Experts say that every two hours spent sitting cuts blood flow, raises blood sugar and reduces 'good' cholesterol levels. A series of studies has linked prolonged sitting to an increased risk of heart disease, diabetes, dementia, obesity and cancer, with one report claiming that sitting for eight hours a day raises your risk of heart disease, cancer and diabetes by 40 per cent.[1]

More recently, a survey of 8,000 people over the age of 45 found that sitting for more than three hours a day results in a significantly increased risk of mortality.[2] Another study links sitting for more than two hours with significantly raised blood pressure.[3]

Prolonged sitting has also been linked to a greater risk of walking disability later in life. A study of 134,000 people over ten years found that those who sat the longest were the least able to walk later on. For this cohort much of the sitting time was spent watching TV, prompting the lead researcher to say, 'TV viewing is a very potent risk factor for disability in older age ... Watching TV for long periods (especially in the evening) has got to be one of the most dangerous things that older people can do because they are much more susceptible to the damages of physical inactivity.'[4]

As if this wasn't enough, a recent study reported that long periods of sitting can also affect our brains, causing thinning in the region of the brain critical for the formation of memories and so perhaps acting as a precursor to Alzheimer's disease.[5]

Although we can all turn off our screens in the evenings, sitting for a mere three hours a day is impossible for those of us in sedentary jobs. But it's not all bad news – and there are things we can do. Researchers found that reducing sitting time – if only slightly – had an immediate impact on mortality rates. Even modest reductions – 10 per cent, for example – seemed to have an instant impact. Another study found that walking for two minutes every hour cut mortality risk by 33 per cent. Best of all, a large study of British women found that fidgeting helped to counter the dangers of sitting for long periods. Those who fidgeted as they sat faced no greater risks of ill health.[6]

The message is clear: cut your daily sitting time, make sure you move after every 30 minutes, and keep fidgeting.

Too sedentary: we say

- Set a timer for 30 minutes and stand up/move for a couple of minutes when it rings.
- Analyse your daily sitting time, then cut it: have walking or standing meetings; work at a standing desk for some of your day; watch TV from an exercise bike; arrange social activities that involve movement.
- Pin a note to your computer screen saying: 'Sitting can kill you'.
- Don't replace sitting with standing. Medics say that this can be just as bad. Replace sitting with moving, even if it's only chair exercises.

- Get up to take or make calls.
- Fidget as you work: we tap our feet, wiggle our knees, shrug our shoulders. Anything goes!
- Invest in a walking desk. Or – cheaper still – buy a set of pedals to put under your desk so that you can pedal as you work. Pedal exercisers start at £15.00 as we write.

High-intensity interval training

In our jobs we spend long periods of time with our backsides welded to our chairs and our eyes fixed to our screens. Indeed, it was partly this that prompted our Project. We knew we had to exercise and yet we had very little free time. High-intensity interval training (HIIT) was one of the most significant discoveries in our Age-Well Project. Indeed, when it comes to ageing, HIIT might be the most beneficial form of exercise you can do. Don't let the word HIIT deter you, because although the name's off-putting, HIIT (sometimes just referred to as HIT – high-intensity training) means nothing more than a short burst of intense activity, followed by a more leisurely pace and then repeated. Sports scientists compare it to the movement of our hunter–gatherer forebears and to the way in which children play, arguing that our bodies were designed to move in bursts of intense activity. And now, a growing body of evidence suggests exercising like this has a more profound effect on our brains, bodies and guts than we once envisaged.[7]

A study published in the publication *Cell Metabolism* found that HIIT increased mitochondrial activity, a cellular process that provides us with energy but declines with age. What intrigued researchers was that the group aged 65–80 experienced a 69 per cent boost in mitochondrial capacity while a younger group had only a 49 per cent boost, leading them to conclude that: 'Vigorous exercise remains the most effective way to bolster health.'[8]

A study published in the *Journal of Cognitive Neuroscience* found that people practising 20 minutes of HIIT a day for only six weeks significantly improved their memories and raised their levels of brain-derived neurotrophic factor (BDNF, as explained on page 44), prompting the lead researcher to suggest that 'as we reach our senior years, we might expect to see even greater benefits in individuals with memory impairment brought on by conditions such as dementia'.[9]

One of the best things about HIIT is its efficiency. Because it takes so little time, we're less likely to avoid it – which makes it an exercise programme that can be sustained over time. A study of sedentary men found that those who trained using a version of HIIT over a period of 12 weeks improved their fitness to the *same levels* and within a *fifth* of the time as a peer group who trained using a traditional model of one hour of continuous movement.[10]

Which is why we like HIIT. We both took up HIIT in our fifties after a thorough investigation into its efficacy and safety. We do 10–20 minute sessions three times a week: Annabel likes rowing and uphill walking, whereas Susan prefers structured classes at the gym. But you can incorporate HIIT into a short jog or even a bike commute because it involves nothing more than going at your usual pace for two minutes, then speeding up for 10–20 seconds until you're out of breath, then reverting to your usual pace for another two minutes, and then speeding up again. Continue this pattern for 10 minutes and do this three times a week. That's it!

HIIT: we say

- Always start slowly and build up intensity over time.
- HIIT can be included in your existing exercise programme. If you walk or cycle regularly, try adding in 20 seconds of extra-fast walking/cycling at certain points (until you become out of breath or sweaty), before returning to your usual speed.
- Don't embark on a new HIIT exercise programme without consulting your doctor first.
- We like to combine short bursts of HIIT with the occasional 'long and slow': a long, steady weekend hike or a cycle ride, for example.

The simple act of walking can change your life

Walking is the easiest, most convenient form of exercise. It's free, requires no equipment, can be done socially or alone and, best of all, it can be squeezed into the busiest of lives. It's also effective: low impact, calorie burning and aerobic. For us, walking was an essential part of our Age-Well Project. We replaced inactive holidays with hiking holidays, Annabel invested in a walking desk, and we bought pedometers and stuck zealously to our minimum of 10,000 steps a day. Our enthusiasm extended to our families, even Annabel's husband swapped his bus commute for a daily seven-mile walk.

Can walking really help you live longer? The science says it can: a recent report in the *American Journal of Preventative*

Medicine found that a regular walking routine can indeed lengthen your life. Researchers looked at data on nearly 140,000 older adults and examined the exercise they'd done during the preceding 13 years. The inactive were 26 per cent more likely to die during the study period than those who walked for up to two hours a week. People who walked for more than two hours a week lowered their risk still further. The researchers think that this is because walking lowers cholesterol and blood pressure levels as well as reducing the risk of heart disease, cancer and diabetes.[11] A 2018 study confirmed this, finding that those who walked as part of their commute cut their risk of dying from heart disease or stroke by 24 per cent.[12]

It's not just our bodies that are protected by regular walking. It appears that our brains benefit too. Using ultrasound to measure blood velocity, and arterial diameters to determine blood flow, researchers found that walking sends pressure waves surging through the arteries, increasing blood to the brain. Running does the same thing (only better), but not cycling, suggesting that the magic lies in the foot-to-ground impact. The researchers also found that walking increases the presence of the protein in the brain we met in Chapter 1, called brain-derived neurotrophic factor (BDNF), prompting the lead researcher to recommend a 30-minute walk five times a week to fend off dementia.[13]

Walk more, walk faster, walk uphill

A stroll has few of the benefits of a brisk walk, however. Which is why we've worked hard to increase our pace over the last few years. A study of 444 older adults found that those with a slower walking speed had a greater risk of developing dementia.[14]

Another study found that people already suffering from heart disease spent less time in hospital if their walking pace was faster.[15] The message? Increase your speed.

It's the speed, the effort, that matters most. Not how long you walk for, which is good news for busy mid-lifers like us, because who can't squeeze in a few short bursts of walking each day? We gleaned this from a new study showing that exertion mattered more than time. In other words, a 10-minute fast walk is more beneficial than a 30-minute meander. 'Despite confusing messages,' said the report's author, 'new research shows all moderate or vigorous activity – even when done in short bursts throughout the day – can reduce the risk of disease and death.'[16] We call this exercise snacking.

If you want to walk vigorously (which means being out of breath and sweaty), nothing beats walking briskly uphill. The best way to do this is to hike in the mountains. Unsurprisingly, most Blue Zoners live in mountainous regions where uphill walking is part of their everyday life. For the rest of us, a treadmill on an incline or a local hill will have to do. Brisk uphill walking burns 60 per cent more calories than brisk walking on the flat, and the American Council on Exercise calls it one of the best exercises for burning fat and shaping muscles. Start gently, as uphill walking puts additional strain on calves and your Achilles tendon.

Walk well – an expert's view

Before you begin walking in earnest, make sure your walking technique is tiptop. We took guidance from a walking instructor, and this is what we learnt: shoulders back and down, head up so you're looking straight ahead, arms loose and swinging like pendulums, bottom tucked in and back straight, abdominals held gently, roll from the heel through the foot so that the heel pushes off. Play around until you feel comfortable. And always wear good supportive footwear.

Walking: we say

- Find walking opportunities throughout the day: take the stairs rather than the lift or add a stretch of walking to your commute.
- If your work is very sedentary, think about investing in a treadmill desk. Annabel wrote a third of this book at a walking desk. If your boss needs convincing, show her the research from Stanford University that discovered walkers are more creative.
- Try a hiking holiday in the hills or add uphill walking to your gym routine.
- Need a walking buddy? www.ramblers.org.uk offers a wide range of group walking activities from short walks to full-scale hiking holidays.
- Wear a pedometer (or use your phone as one). We swear by ours – not only do they remind us to move, but they also track our steps over time, enabling us to constantly challenge ourselves. We now clock over 100,000 steps a week – much of it by stealth (commuting, shopping, dog-walking, school runs, gardening, and so on).
- Check your walking technique (see above) and invest in comfortable flat shoes or trainers.

- Still struggling? Try an app – the best ones track speed, distance, incline and all-day steps. We recently trialled MapMyWalk, Walkmeter App and Argus, but there are plenty of others, including some that donate to charity. www.verywellfit.com runs regular reviews of walking apps and pedometers.
- Feeling down? Take a walk somewhere green. Research suggests that a walk in nature can reduce anxiety and depression.[17]
- Use walking poles for support or for an upper body workout. We use walking poles on long hikes for better balance, greater stability and to keep our upper body and core working. Research suggests that walking with poles burns more calories – if that's your aim.[18]
- Carry a backpack rather than a handbag. Ideally, have your belongings in your pocket, but we know that isn't always practical!

Spend time with trees

Trees are good for our stress, our blood pressure, our memory and more. In the last decade, scientists have begun uncovering the powerful effects of trees. Not only for the environment or the landscape, but also for human health. Simply put, being among trees can do wonders for our health.

A psychologist at Western Michigan University, Roger Ulrich, spearheaded some of the earliest studies into the effects of nature. He found that people who viewed nature photos after being exposed to a stressful task reported increased feelings of affection, friendliness, and happiness. The group that viewed urban scenes reported feeling sad. Since then, researchers have found that recovering patients who look on to trees need less pain relief and leave hospital earlier than those looking at a wall. Housing estates with visible green space report less domestic violence, and blood pressure falls within three minutes of being in green space.[19]

Japan has pioneered and funded the most ambitious studies. Here, spending time in trees is known as *shinrin-yoku*, which translates as 'forest bathing'. Between 2004 and 2014, the Japanese government spent $4 million studying the impact of forest bathing. Researchers discovered that forest bathing:

- Lowered rates of the stress hormone cortisol.
- Lowered blood pressure.
- Lowered the heart rate.
- Boosted immunity.
- Significantly lowered blood glucose levels in older people with type-2 diabetes.
- Cut levels of anxiety, anger and depression, and improved energy levels.

A mere fifteen minutes was all it took. But how long did the effects last? A team from Nippon Medical School found that forest visits had a long-lasting influence on immune-system markers, increasing the activity of antiviral cells and intracellular anti-cancer proteins – changes that remained significant for an entire week after the visit. Meanwhile, a weekend of forest bathing was found to have positive effects on immunity that lasted up to a month.[20]

Researchers think that the power of trees might lie in the chemicals they secrete, called phytoncides. Phytoncides are produced by trees and plants to protect themselves from harmful germs, and are particularly prevalent in pine and fir trees. A more recent theory speculates that it's the microbes (specifically *Mycobacterium vaccae*) found in forest soil that makes us feel better. When researchers injected this harmless bacteria into mice, they found the mice behaving as if they'd taken antidepressants. *Mycobacterium vaccae* also appears to activate neurons associated with immunity.[21]

Can being among trees also help our brains? Research has shown that cortisol adversely affects our brains, damaging the prefrontal cortex and hippocampus.[22] If forest bathing reduces cortisol, this can only benefit our brains.

Research has also been conducted on the relationship between trees and memory. Marc Berman, a neuroscientist at the University of Michigan, sent out groups of walkers and then measured their short-term memory. Those walking in trees improved their memory by 20 per cent, whereas those walking in urban areas showed no improvement, suggesting that regular woodland walks could have benefits for those suffering from mild cognitive impairment.[23]

It's not only memory that's improved by a walk in the wild. Sleep has also been shown to improve following an afternoon 'green' walk. A Japanese study found that people taking a two-hour afternoon walk in woodland slept for almost an hour longer at night.[24] A further study compared urban and green walks of approximately 17 minutes in duration and found that the 'green' walks resulted in an additional 20 minutes of sleep compared to the urban walks.[25] Interestingly, morning walks didn't have the same effect.

Tree 'therapy': we say

- Investigate local forest and woodlands that offer weekends or holiday breaks, like Forest Holidays in the UK (www.forestholidays.co.uk) or Eco Retreats in Wales (www.ecoretreats.co.uk).
- Find your nearest woodland and walk there regularly.
- If you have surplus land or garden, plant a tree.
- Don't just 'bathe', walk!
- Try an afternoon walk in woodland or your local park to improve your sleep.

Exercise to improve your bone density

Exercise doesn't just build muscle – it builds bone too. Our bones are constantly rebuilding and remodelling themselves, adapting to whatever comes their way – including exercise, or inactivity. When we move, gravity and muscle contraction impact our bones: the old adage, use it or lose it, is never truer than when it comes to bone strength. Research has shown that professional tennis players have much higher bone density in their serving arm than their non-serving arm.[26]

There are at least 200 million people around the world with osteoporosis, and millions more who suffer frailty and fractures as a result of bones weakening with age. Therefore, finding the right exercise to strengthen our bones, before it's too late, is critical.

Researchers from the University of São Paolo in Brazil

crunched through all the existing data on the impact of exercise on bone density to find the exercise most beneficial to post-menopausal women:[27]

The best bone-strengthening exercise of all time

- **Jump** Yes, really. Jumping 10 to 20 times a day with 30 seconds of rest between each jump provides greater bone-building benefits than running or jogging, according to the research.[28]

The really good ones

- **High-impact exercise** In one study, women who were given a six-month regime of high-impact exercise (running, jumping, skipping etc.) showed a greater increase in bone density than women who did weight training.
- **Resistance training** Multiple studies show that dynamic resistance training, for example, lifting weights, is beneficial for bones, and exerts less pressure on joints than high-impact exercise.
- **Trampolining and t'ai chi** Both improve proprioception (no, we hadn't heard of it either): the connection between sensation and movement. Exercises that improve our awareness of what our bodies are doing result in better postural control, mobility and a reduced incidence of falls.
- **Dance**, especially ballroom dancing, also improves proprioception, as well as balance, coordination and cognition, resulting in fewer falls.

Worth a try

- **Walking** is good for the thigh bones of post-menopausal women, but it doesn't help build strength in the spine.
- **Running** A study found that runners over 65 had better total bone density than a control group.
- **Swimming and aquarobics** are not the best exercises for building bone mass (as they're not weight bearing) *but* researchers found that swimmers had a higher bone turn-over and, therefore, stronger bones than a control group of non-exercisers. Water-based exercise is particularly good for people struggling with high-impact fitness.

Not so good

- **Cycling** It's terrific exercise, but it *doesn't* build bone strength. In fact, professional cyclists tend to have lower bone mass density and higher fracture risk due to the lack of weight-bearing movement while exercising.

Exercise and bone health: we say

- Jump! We incorporate jumping exercises into our gym routines. Try burpees – they're a killer, but effective. Or simply jump on and off a low box. Our gym has 30cm mats that we leap on and off.
- Wear good trainers – well tied. It sounds obvious, but tie your shoelaces for better support.
- Warm up, and cool down, properly. If you don't stretch

after a workout, the chances of injury are greatly
increased.
- We work on our cores for overall strength and stability.
Yoga, Pilates and stretching all help.

Be aware that the National Osteoporosis Society advises that
if you have a high fracture risk, and particularly if you've
had fragility fractures (including compression fractures in the
spine), sudden new high-impact exercise (jogging, jumping,
and so on) are best avoided. Exercise advice needs to be tai-
lored to your own needs, so discuss this with your doctor or
physiotherapist.

Work with weights

Weights? Resistance training? Isn't that for gym bunnies or
budding bodybuilders? Yes, we thought so, too. We envisaged
our mid-life enjoying gentle yoga classes or strolling in the park.
But talk to any expert on longevity and it becomes crystal clear:
resistance training is as important as aerobic exercise, eating
vegetables and getting a good night's sleep.

Every week that we fail to build muscle, we increase our
chances of getting osteoporosis. After the age of 40, we lose bone
mass at the rate of 1 per cent a year. A study from the University
of Buffalo found that women who hadn't done resistance training
were much more likely to become dangerously frail, prompting
the lead researcher to urge women to build muscle strength early
in the ageing process.[29] Think of it as building your strength and

endurance reserves. The happy by-product is toned, honed limbs, the ability to lift and carry more, and better quality sleep. Texas University found that six months of resistance training improved the sleep quality of 70-year-olds by 38 per cent – in addition to reversing the adverse effects of hormone loss and halting the decrease of blood flow to ageing legs.[30]

We also know that strength training can reduce the risk of heart attacks, heart disease, strokes and type-2 diabetes, as well as slowing bone loss and easing the pain of arthritis. A study in the *Journal of Preventive Medicine* found that older adults who did strength training at least twice a week had 46 per cent lower odds of death from all causes, a 41 per cent lower risk of cardiac death and 19 per cent lower risk of dying from cancer, than those who did no strength training.[31]

We'd never worked with free weights before (too intimidating, too dull), but our research into ageing convinced us that working with our own body weight and a pair of hand weights was the most efficient, convenient way to build strength. Unlike machines, which often work a single isolated muscle, working with weights and your own body can build multiple muscles in one go while simultaneously improving your balance. It's also considerably more convenient.

We put pairs of weights strategically round our homes: in the kitchen beside the kettle; in the bathroom next to the sink; in front of the TV. Every time we brewed a cup of tea, we spent a couple of minutes doing bicep curls, shoulder presses, tricep presses and lateral raises. After cleaning our teeth we did a few squats. If we watched TV, we lunged with weights. Not always, of course. But enough to see the benefits.

Eventually we added dead weights, tricep dips, push-ups and abdominal crunches along with other floor exercises recommended by the trainers at our gym or that we unearthed in books or on YouTube. You don't need weights when you start – you can use books, bottles of water or cans of beans. If you're serious, however, invest in a set of graded hand weights (2, 3 and 4kg are the only weights we use, doubling them up when need be). We'd always recommend asking a professional to look over your technique. When starting out, use a mirror, join a class or invest in a personal training session.

By doing resistance training in bite-sized 'snacks' using 'dead' time, we became stronger almost by stealth. It's not necessary to weight-train in lengthy blocks. The important thing is to squeeze a little into your life, and the sooner the better. In the summer we take our weights outside, thereby killing two birds with one stone: getting vitamin D and sunlight while building muscle. If you're lucky enough to have an out-door fitness centre in your local park, use it.

How much weight training should we do? A new study says that an hour a week will reduce our risk of heart attack and stroke by 40–70 per cent and anything above this has no additional benefit. All it takes, therefore, is less than nine minutes a day. Nor does this need to be done with weights. As the author of this report said, 'Muscles don't know the difference between digging the yard, carrying heavy shopping bags or lifting a dumbbell.'[32]

If you travel frequently, consider buying a resistance band. These lightweight elastic bands slip into the most crammed of suitcases and come with simple strength-building exercises that can be done anywhere, at any time. On this note, we'll share our top tip: don't worry about what other people think or about making an idiot of yourself. We do calf raises while standing on the tube, squats while waiting at the bus stop and lunges while standing in queues. Our children squirm with embarrassment, but so what?

Don't forget the importance of variety. The human body contains 640 muscles, so to stand a chance of exercising even 20 per cent of these, we need to mix up our strength-training exercises. If boredom kicks in, try rope climbing, climbing walls or boot-camp classes. We swear by rowing, which combines strength and aerobic training, uses 85 per cent of our muscles across nine major muscle groups and burns around 300 calories an hour.

- Don't delay – start building muscle today.
- Invest in a set of hand weights.
- If your time is very limited, focus on your upper body (unless you're entirely sedentary), as the muscles in your lower body are worked as you walk, run and cycle.
- Work out in sunlight if possible.
- Mix and match to reach as many muscles/muscle groups as possible.
- Find a buddy to keep you motivated. Research shows that people working out with a partner have a greater chance of sticking with it.
- Use dead time to work those muscles and don't give a damn what passers-by think!

Dance – shake your booty

We already know about the extraordinary power of exercise to improve the brain in older people. Regular exercise – whatever it is – is good for us, protecting our brains as well as our bodies.

But not all exercise is equal. And when it comes to fending off cognitive decline, dancing is the queen bee of exercise.

Not all dancing is equal, though. To enjoy the full brain-and-body benefits of dance, you need a dance programme that works the brain as hard as it works the body. This means regularly learning new steps and routines: ballroom dancing, modern dance, Scottish dancing, line-dancing, Zumba, jazz and disco-dancing all fit the bill. The trick is to keep learning new routines, as you move, rather than working repeatedly on the same old choreography. Simply perfecting one routine has been proven to have no effect on the brain.

Researchers at the German Centre for Neurodegenerative Diseases ran an 18-month programme in which they compared the brain effects of standard endurance training (cycling and walking) with dancing, in a group of elderly men and women. The dancers participated in twice-weekly 90-minute classes for the first six months, followed by a single weekly class for the next six months. In all classes they were exposed to constantly changing choreographies, which they had to memorise. The researchers found that both groups showed an increase in the hippocampus region of the brain (that's the part associated with memory and learning) but the dancers showed the largest increase and the most improved balance.[33]

The Albert Einstein College of Medicine found similar results in a 21-year study investigating the effects of 11 different activities, including cycling, golf, swimming and tennis. The researchers concluded that dance significantly lowered participants' risk of dementia – by a huge 76 per cent. Again, the participants were doing freestyle dance in which they had to make constant, split-second decisions about how, where and when to move. The study's author attributed the 76 per cent reduction in dementia risk to the combined triple whammy of benefits: social interaction, an aerobic workout and a powerful cognitive boost. Ballroom dancing is, perhaps, the most social dancing of all, forcing you to interact with others.

Other studies have found Zumba to improve mood and cognitive skills,[34] and Scottish dancing to reduce age-related decline in women over the age of 70.[35]

As we researched this book, we experimented with a variety of dance classes, from disco to ballet, from Regency to ballroom. What we love about dance is the way it combines a brain and body workout with social interaction, thereby ticking several Age-Well boxes in one go. More importantly, it's great fun.

Dance: we say

- Introduce a dance class (or two or three) into your exercise programme.
- Vary your classes and dance styles, and make sure your teacher changes the routines frequently.
- Concentrate as hard as you can. As soon as you stop focusing, the brain stops working.
- It's not just about the classes: go dancing, socially, in the evenings.
- Dance with different partners – if you become used to the same partner your brain won't work as hard.
- Start now. The best time to begin building your cognitive reserve is as soon as possible.
- No classes near you? Use YouTube to teach yourself, or find a freelance dance teacher and set up a class in your local church hall.

A rowing machine might be your body's best friend

When we started our Age-Well Project, we had bingo wings.
The underside of our upper arms were beginning to droop,
much to the hilarity of our children. Since then, however, we've
discovered every woman's answer to bingo wings, and ours are
long gone. More significantly, we've discovered that the best
exercise for bingo wings just happens to be the best exercise for
your heart.

We know that exercise must include vigour: studies consistently rate high-intensity interval training (HIIT) as one of the
best and most efficient ways to delay ageing and improve cardiovascular fitness, as we saw earlier in this chapter.

But once you've decided to squeeze some HIIT into your exercise programme, what should you do? Run? Cycle? Stair-climb?
We're always on the lookout for highly efficient exercise, low-
impact activities that involve the entire body and that combine
strength training with vigorous aerobic exercise. We particularly
like activities that are HIIT-friendly, meaning that we can easily
adjust speed and effort.

Which is why we love rowing. The rowing machines in
our gym are always unused, with a forlorn lonely look about
them. But the research speaks for itself: rowing is hugely efficient, particularly if you adopt HIIT principles (20 seconds
of fast rowing followed by 1–2 minutes of slower rowing).
According to Peta Bee and Dr Sarah Schenker, authors of
The Ageless Body, rowing is 'second to none in improving
cardiovascular fitness'.[36] Ask any personal trainer, and they'll
tell you that rowing is the most effective form of exercise for
a full body workout. Studies comparing rowing with cycling
support this.[37]

Why? Because rowing works 84 per cent of the muscles in your body and all the major muscle groups – including the calves, quads, hamstrings, glutes, abdominals, obliques, pectorals, biceps, triceps, deltoids, core, lower and middle back – in one fell swoop. For us, this means a cardiovascular workout that simultaneously builds body-wide strength. Even the tiny muscles in our wrists are worked when we row. And that means less time doing weight-training.

Rowing can do more than dispense with bingo wings. According to John Gibbons, osteopath for the Oxford University rowing team, rowing helps prevent osteoporosis by strengthening bones. He says the range of gripping, pulling, extending and bending movements stimulates the production of bone-forming cells, which increase bone-mass density. And, unlike running, he says, rowing is gentle on the joints.[38]

To get the best results, you need the right technique. Ask a personal trainer or rower to watch your technique. Alternatively look on YouTube or visit www.concept2.com, which contains a wealth of information on technique.

We use machines in the local gym, but our friends who do genuine river rowing glean the extra benefits of fresh air, sunlight and social interaction.

Rowing: we say

- Most gyms have rowing machines that are rarely used. Ten minutes two to three times a week is enough for visible results within a few weeks.
- If you're not a gym-goer and have no nearby river, British Rowing holds Go Row classes for beginners.

- Alternatively, invest in a rowing machine (these aren't cheap but they can be picked up second-hand, although they are impractically large).

Play table tennis

You might not believe this, but ping-pong could be the single most effective sport when it comes to fending off dementia. *Alzheimer's Weekly* reported a clear increase in motor skills and cognitive awareness from playing ping-pong, after clinical studies in Japan found it markedly increased blood flow to the brain. 'The clear increase in motor skills and cognitive awareness from playing table tennis is significant, if not remarkable, in its unique benefits for brain disease patients,' the journal stated.[39]

Another Japanese study found that regularly playing ping-pong not only lowered the risk of dementia but could stabilise and even improve symptoms in those already presenting with cognitive impairment. More recently, a Taiwanese report found that six months of table tennis uniquely enhanced cognition, opening up different neurological pathways from those generated by walking.[40]

Unlike jogging or swimming, for example, table tennis stimulates many different parts of the brain. When Dr Matthew Kempton ran a study comparing the brains of walkers and ping-pong players over ten weeks, he found that both groups had more neurons in the hippocampus than those who did neither, but that the ping-pong players showed an increase in the thickness of their cortex – the part of the brain associated with complex thinking and the part which shrinks most as we age.[41]

Professor of Neuroscience and author of *Healthy Brain, Happy Life*, Wendy Suzuki, agrees. 'There's a lot going on in table tennis: attention is increasing, memory is increasing, you have a better mood. And you're building motor circuits in your brain. A bigger part of your brain is being activated.'[42] She points out, however, that to get the full benefits you need to be playing fast ping-pong (so that's probably not with a beer in one hand and half an eye on the TV).

Table tennis isn't only good for the brain. It also improves hand–eye co-ordination and provides an aerobic workout that involves both the upper and lower body. As Lisa Feldermann, personal training programme manager at Blink Fitness in New York, said:

Most table tennis beginners burn between 200–350 calories an hour … but elite competitors burn up to 500 calories per match. It's a total body sport … quads, calves and hip abductors are all hard at work, also forearms, obliques, abdominals, biceps, shoulders and triceps as well as stabilising muscles like the rhomboids and middle trapezius.[43]

Ping-pong is easy on the joints, improves reflexes, and is very social (particularly so as it can be played by almost anyone, at any age, from any background, making it a very democratic sport). It requires no expensive kit, membership or lessons, it can be played indoors or outdoors, and it uses very little space.

A study from Oxford University, which attempted to tease out the sports most likely to increase longevity, found racket sports – namely tennis and badminton – reduced the risk of death at any given age by 50 per cent, well ahead of football or running, and even ahead of dance and swimming.[44] The study didn't include table tennis, but we think if it had, the sport would have featured alongside other racket sports. We're big fans of table tennis. We love its convenience, its simplicity and the sheer fun of it.

Table tennis: we say

- Our local park has table tennis tables. See if yours does. Or visit https://www.pingengland.co.uk/.
- To join a club, visit https://tabletennisengland. co.uk/ or http://ttwwebsite.co.uk/ (Wales) or http:// tabletennisscotland.co.uk/ or http://www.irishtabletennis. com/. Note: many have teams for over fifties or older people.
- Or do as we did: treat yourself to a fold-up table, keep it open and play with whoever's around.
- We love Bounce, the chain of bars combining eating, drinking, dancing and ping-pong, set up by a former competitive table-tennis player. Bounce (only in London and Chicago at the time of writing) hosts informal tournaments, ladies nights, LGBT nights and more: www. bouncepingpong.com.

Yoga

The fact that yoga has been credited with improving 101 health conditions, from Alzheimer's to urinary incontinence,[45] should be enough to entice anyone into downward-facing dog – it certainly worked for us. Yoga, and its Chinese cousins, t'ai chi and qi gong, have also been found to aid longevity. They all combine breath, movement and meditation. And all three have been found to increase the activity of telomerase, the enzyme that keeps our telomeres long (as explained in Chapter 1).[46, 47]

Take any yoga, t'ai chi or qi gong class and you'll quickly understand how the stretching and balancing exercises ease many of the physical ailments associated with ageing: back pain, stiff joints, failing balance and muscle loss. We've both suffered back pain and were intrigued by research comparing the benefits of general exercise to those of Iyengar yoga – which focuses on body alignment – for lower back-pain sufferers. It found that while general exercise reduced pain by over 40 per cent in a six-month period, the yoga practitioners saw a 70 per cent reduction.[48]

Mind–body interventions, such as yoga, t'ai chi and qi gong, work at a cellular level too: they appear to reduce the risk of inflammatory conditions. When the body is under stress – in 'fight or flight' mode – genes produce proteins called cytokines, which cause inflammation, accelerated ageing and a higher risk of cancer. These practices reduce pro-inflammatory gene expression so that fewer cytokines are produced.[49]

It's no surprise that the combination of physical exercise and stress reduction is hugely beneficial for those with cardiovascular disease. A meta-analysis of yoga's impact on hypertension found that the practice effectively reduced blood pressure.[50] And oxidative stress, which lies at the heart of much disease, is reduced by doing yoga: in tests on men aged 60–80 yoga was found to increase levels of antioxidants.[51]

Yoga's impact on the brain is as powerful as that on the body. It can reduce the symptoms of depression: US Army veterans who took part in twice-weekly yoga sessions reported a significant reduction in depressive symptoms after eight weeks. A further study found that yoga significantly reduced depressive symptoms in people not on antidepressants, or for whom antidepressants weren't working.[52]

Research suggests that yoga can improve symptoms of mild cognitive impairment (MCI), often a precursor to Alzheimer's. In one study, middle-aged people with MCI showed improvement in visuospatial and verbal memory after 12 weeks of yoga.[53] Further studies on healthy, older brains after yoga practice show increases in grey matter in the central nervous system, amygdala (the seat of our emotions) and frontal cortex (the part of our brain responsible for planning and decision making).[54] Similar research on elderly t'ai chi practitioners found that they had increased brain volume after eight months, compared to a control group.[55] Dementia patients on a movement course combining yoga, t'ai chi, qi gong and dance showed improvement in memory recall and learnt to anticipate the physical movements associated with each piece of music.[56] The study, called 'Happy Antics', was conducted in association with the Alzheimer's Society. Wouldn't it be wonderful to see a programme like this available to all dementia sufferers?

Yoga: we say

- If it sounds too 'hippy dippy', try gentle stretching. It'll help with muscle remodelling, connective-tissue strengthening, range-of-motion improvement, joint alignment and potentially blood flow. Many of the elders we interviewed for this book had their own stretching routines. Find one on YouTube.

- If you're time pressed, take a class then practise at home. Alternatively, download a yoga app or find a class you like on YouTube.

- If you have osteopenia or osteoporosis, talk to your doctor before starting any new exercise.

- Make sure you have comfortable clothes and a non-slip yoga mat.

Staying Engaged

In this section we explore the science of staying socially and intellectually engaged and we examine the attitudinal traits associated with longevity. According to geroscientists and researchers, staying involved and actively engaged with life is one of the markers of healthy ageing. As ever, teasing out cause and effect isn't easy. But all too often those enjoying the longest, least diseased lives are those with the busiest lives.

In a nutshell: spend time with friends and family; make new friends; look after your partner; do anything that keeps you in touch with others, from volunteering to walking a dog with a neighbour. We can learn from SuperAgers,[1] who typically have extensive social networks. Some neuroscientists think that having a large social network might be a vital catalyst for keeping our brains and bodies in great shape: older people with larger social networks often have better cognition, better mortality rates, and better survival rates post-heart attack.[2] Meanwhile, social isolation is linked to a 32 per cent higher risk of stroke, a 40 per cent greater risk of dementia[3] and a 29 per cent higher risk of heart disease.[4] It's also linked to a greater risk of inflammation, depression and all-cause mortality. Small wonder that some medics and psychologists believe staying socially engaged is the single most important thing we can do to age well.

Staying socially engaged is enhanced and complemented by staying intellectually engaged.

For years, scientists assumed that we had a finite number of irreplaceable brain cells, as is the case with rodents and primates. We now know this isn't true. New research shows that we continue making brain cells (neurons) until we die – if we look after our brains, that is. Not only can we constantly replenish neurons, but we can also make them at the same rate and in the same quantity – although perhaps not of the same quality – as any young person.

Neuroscientists are still untangling the astonishing complexities of the brain. But one thing is clear: our brains can be as sharp – if not sharper – in our old age as they were in the heady days of our youth. The most important factors in maintaining a blade-sharp brain are: physical exercise; keeping the brain stimulated by reading, learning and working; embracing novelty to keep our neurons firing; avoiding stress, depression and excess alcohol; eating a good diet with plenty of omega-3s; staying socially engaged; and getting quality sleep. In this section we also show you the best ways to keep your brain rewiring (and, no, it's not a daily crossword).

Also in this section we examine the science of attitude. Longevity researchers are increasingly discovering a unique personality profile among the very long-lived, a particular set of character traits that any of us can adopt and hone. These include a strong sense of purpose, high levels of resilience, a *positive attitude to growing old, a propensity for laughter, and a profound sense of gratitude often (but not always) expressed through faith. These traits, it seems, can enable us to recover more quickly from illness and trauma as well as contributing to the stamina sometimes necessary to carry on living long after your peers.*

CHAPTER 8

Stay Social

We both live in very busy households, where family, friends, neighbours and pets come and go. To boot, Susan's work involves a constant stream of meetings in a buzzy Central London office, and even Annabel's relatively solitary life as a writer involves plenty of communication with editors, agents and publicists. For us, a couple of days with nothing but our own company is utter bliss.

Our busy lives bode well for our long-term health. But we're very aware that our days won't always be as bustling as they are now. And research makes it clear that social connection is a biological need, almost as important as food or sleep.

As for the previous Cornerstones, our 'We Say' boxes in this and the following chapters include numerous suggestions to help you stay engaged. We hope one or two (or more) will tempt you to learn something new or try something different. For an overview, see also our brief explanation of the staying engaged section in the Introduction.

Sharing, caring, community and humanity matter

With all the endless – and satisfyingly scientific – news on diet, sleep and exercise, it's easy to overlook the role of social support in longevity. But this would be a *big mistake.* According to the UK's Royal College of GPs, the 1.2 million Britons thought to be suffering from loneliness are 50 per cent more likely to die prematurely, making loneliness as big a mortality risk as diabetes.[1] This reflects several studies linking the health impact of loneliness and social isolation to dementia, heart disease, stroke, depression and a 29 per cent greater risk of dying.[2, 3]

Meanwhile, other reports found that cancer and heart-attack patients with the largest number of friends made the best recoveries. A meta-analysis of 148 studies of heart-attack patients found that having a good support network was as good a predictor of survival as giving up smoking.

Without a robust social network, our lives are not only emptier but more prone to ill health. Psychology Professor Julianne Holt-Lunstad believes that when it comes to healthy ageing, loneliness and social isolation are as bad for our health as smoking, air pollution and obesity.[4, 5]

Many believe that we're now living through a loneliness epidemic, exacerbated by social trends that include smaller households, higher rates of childlessness, less religious faith, longer working hours and a more transient workforce. This is the very opposite of what happens in the Blue Zones where people tend to live in the same neighbourhood all their lives, often with other family members, as well as going to church and regularly socialising. Longevity researcher Susan Pinker believes that close personal relationships and social cohesion lie at the nub of Blue Zone longevity.[6]

To better understand the link between socialising and longevity, we turned to a landmark eight-decade study that began in 1921 and continued into this century. In this vast bank of data Drs Friedman and Martin found a clear correlation between having a large social network and living longer. Interestingly, they found no correlation between *feeling* loved or cared for and longevity. It was the *size* of social network that mattered most. More recent research has added to this, suggesting that it's also the *quality* of our friendships: do our friends stimulate us? Do they have a positive outlook?

The second most significant correlation with longevity was helping and caring for others. Therefore, those who played a supportive role in multiple networks reaped the Age-Well benefits of helping others and simultaneously being part of a large social network.[7] Volunteering has long been associated with better physical and mental health, including lower rates of mortality and less depression.[8] Last year another study added to the evidence, reporting that volunteers also had better cognition.[9]

With all the attention on good social networks, however, it's easy to overlook the power of small, daily connections from those we don't know. A Canadian study found that the little moments of connection from people we don't consider friends or family ('weak ties') can also make a significant contribution to our happiness and well-being.[10]

Grow your social network Investigate volunteering by visiting https://do-it.org/ – a comprehensive website that lists the opportunities in your area. Or identify your interests and go from there. Interested in crime? The Old Bailey takes volunteers. Love history? The National Trust needs volunteers for its historic homes. Or join a book group, walking group, bridge circle or choir. If there's a U3A (University of the Third Age) in your area, get involved. Local libraries are a good place to sniff out what's happening in your neighbourhood.

Eat with other people A 2018 report from Oxford Economics found that those who always ate with other people had greater well-being and happiness than people who ate alone.[11]

Help create a neighbourhood community Over the years we've held coffee mornings and curry nights, and helped organise street parties and cricket matches. Pay special attention to the milestones that can act as catalysts to isolation and/or loneliness: retirement, divorce, widowhood, ill health and empty-nest syndrome. At these times make sure your diary includes some social occasions, however small.

Use social media to stay in touch Although it can't replicate the emotional depth of being face-to-face, social media is quick, accessible and convenient. A study of 12 million Facebook users found that they outlived non-users, when the site was used to help preserve actual social ties. Those with the largest FB networks also outlived the 10 per cent with the smallest networks.[12] In Wendy Mitchell's poignant account of living with dementia, she writes about the importance of blogging, Facebook and Twitter for maintaining her social network and feeling socially engaged.[13]

Make use of communal spaces and activities: allotments, park ping-pong tables, church choirs. Professors Blackburn and Epel found that people living in communities with low social cohesion had greater cellular ageing and shorter telomeres.[14]

Greet people, strike up conversations, or simply smile. We often do this, even though it mortifies our children.

Many – if not all – the suggestions in this book have the potential to include others, from dancing to meditating, from learning a language to walking, from doing something creative to playing table tennis. To build your social network, always opt for the social version of an activity. Besides, you'll probably have more fun and you're more likely to persist with it.

Should you get married to live longer?

A daft question, of course. No one should marry to live longer, regardless of the occasional headline that pops up in the national press. And yet research has consistently shown that married people appear to have some sort of longevity advantage. Indeed, the findings have been so consistent that researchers now talk of the marriage protection hypothesis.

Let's be clear, though: it's happily married *men* who reap the greatest health advantages from the state of matrimony. In 1921 a man named Dr Terman began studying a cohort of 1,500 American children born around 1910. The study continued for many decades (long after Terman's own death) and eventually became a book that fully analysed and explored every facet of the cohort's lives. The authors found that the longest-living people were usually those they termed the 'steadily marrieds'. Like previous studies, the Terman study found divorced men to have a much higher risk of mortality, with remarried men not far behind.

Single men fared better than both divorced and remarried

men, but not as well as the steadily married men (one study gave steadily married men a 46 per cent lower rate of death).[15] Incidentally, a later study found that men married to highly educated women had an even lower mortality risk.

Women, however, responded differently. Although the 'steadily marrieds' still did best, divorced women didn't lag far behind. Nor did steadily single women. As the authors succinctly put it, 'women who could thrive in a good marriage tended to stay especially healthy, but many of the rest were better off single'.

More recently, doctors from Harvard found that married couples were more likely to identify cancer in the early stages and less likely to die from it,[16] whereas married prostate cancer patients lived almost twice as long as unmarried patients. A meta-analysis published in *Heart* found heart disease less prevalent in married people than in unmarried, divorced or widowed people.[17]

Now it also appears that marriage can help to fend off dementia. A new meta-analysis of 15 studies, involving over 800,000 people from across the world, found that lifelong single people had a 42 per cent elevated risk of dementia compared with their married counterparts.[18] In a *BMJ* podcast the report's author explained that it's not marriage per se that keeps dementia away but the social interaction and greater attention to health that marriage brings.[19]

According to Dr Robert Butler, author of *The Longevity Prescription*, 'it is a statistical fact that a good marriage at age 50 is a better predictor of good health at 80 than a low cholesterol count'. It appears that the emotional, financial, social and practical support that marriage offers might well provide a buffer against some diseases of ageing. Professor Robert Waldinger certainly thinks so. After conducting several studies into the protective power of positive relationships, he summed up with these words: 'Good relationships don't just protect our bodies, they protect our brains ... they don't have to be smooth all the time, so long as one feels they can count on the other when the going gets tough. Tending to your relationships is a form of self-care.'[20]

As 'steadily marrieds' (at the time of writing, that is!) we absorbed the above information and then did a little work on our own affairs (no, we don't mean those sorts of affairs). We're not marriage-guidance counsellors, but we did – occasionally – go out of our way to be extra-specially kind to our other halves, even when we felt tired and grumpy. We also pointed out how indispensable we were to *their* health, thereby encouraging them to reciprocate our little acts of kindness!

If you're single, however, the research findings highlight the importance of having a strong circle of friends, neighbours and extended family to counter social isolation. You should be particularly vigilant about looking after yourself, too, as there'll be no one else nudging or nagging you into exercising more, drinking less or eating more vegetables.

Relationships: we say

We're not relationship experts, but the advice seems to be:

- Tend to your marriage as you'd tend to your health – nurture it in whatever ways work for the both of you.
- Retirement is often a complicated and difficult time for cohabiting/married couples. Experts suggest discussing it in advance and making some sort of a plan to address the sudden 'throwing together' that retirement entails.

Have faith, and find your 'church'

There are few things more personal than the concept of faith. Only you know what you believe, and whether you want to express that belief through some form of religious practice. What we do know, however, is that those with faith appear to live longer.

Several studies have found a consistent link between frequent religious attendance and longevity, even after controlling for other factors. In a meta-analysis involving 126,000 people, those who attended religious services had a 29 per cent chance of living longer. The protective effects were greater for women than men, and greater when religious practice was public rather than private.[21]

An early pioneering study found that men who were weekly churchgoers reduced their risk of dying from heart disease by 40 per cent. A study of 21,000 Americans found those attending a religious service more than once a week had a longer life span by 7 years, doubling to 14 years for African Americans.[22] A survey of over 5,000 people found that churchgoers had lower levels of 'allostatic load' (wear and tear on the body, including blood pressure and cholesterol levels, as a result of chronic stress) than non-churchgoers and were 46 per cent less likely to die during the 18-year follow-up period.[23]

Researchers analysing obituaries found that people who had a religious affiliation while alive lived at least four years longer than those without.[24] The researchers adjusted for the social aspect of religious observance, which added only an extra year of life. They suggest that there might be other explanations: religious believers are less likely to indulge in unhealthy behaviours such as drug and alcohol abuse, plus, they add, 'many religions promote stress-reducing practices that may improve health, such as gratitude, prayer, or meditation'.

Religion has such a powerful impact on the brain that it has its own field of neurological study: neurotheology. Religion activates the same reward-processing brain circuits as sex, drugs and other addictive activities.[25] Engaging in spiritual practices raises levels of endorphins and the 'happiness' neurotransmitter, serotonin. Research shows that both meditating Buddhists and praying Catholic nuns have increased activity in the frontal lobes of the brain, areas that control focus and attention. In his book, *How God Changes Your Brain*, Professor Andrew Newberg details how religious rituals have a positive effect on the brain, even if the spiritual references are removed.

Centenarians practise religion in all of the Blue Zones (the areas of the world with the highest proportion of people living past 100). In *The Blue Zones*, author Dan Buettner says, 'People who pay attention to their spiritual side have lower rates of cardiovascular disease, depression, stress, and suicide, and their immune systems seem to work better ... To a certain extent, adherence to a religion allows them to relinquish the stresses of everyday life to a higher power.'

We find this research intriguing. Even after adjusting for factors such as higher educational attainment and greater opportunity for socialisation, the results suggest that faith contains an elusive something that contributes to longevity. Is it the meditative qualities of prayer? The moment of calm in a hectic week? The exercise required to reach a place of worship? Or something altogether more mystical? Only you can decide.

Religion: we say

- If religion isn't your thing, find your 'church' in other ways. Try the shared euphoria of a sporting event or a music concert.
- Several of the nonagenarians we interviewed for this book observe some form of religious practice. You can read their stories in Chapter 14.
- Find other ways to reap the benefits of religious observance: volunteer, meditate, practise gratitude, socialise.
- Attend your local place of worship, and see how you feel.
- If the faith you were raised in no longer appeals, try another one. Some of the happiest people we know converted to Buddhism as adults.

Working longer will keep you younger

We have no intention of retiring – ever. A bold statement perhaps. And if we become incapacitated, we might be forced into retirement. But it'll be against our will. Why? Firstly, because we enjoy our work – its daily challenges, the social interaction it brings, the opportunities for creativity, the sense of purpose. Secondly, because research tells us that people who work longer age better.

A 2016 study of 2,956 people of retirement age concluded, chillingly, with these words: 'Early retirement may be a risk factor for mortality and prolonged working life may provide survival benefits among US adults.'[26] So much for the dream of retirement!

The study reflected earlier large-scale longitudinal studies indicating that 25 per cent of American retirees[27] and around 10 per cent of German retirees[28] experienced significant reductions in health and well-being following retirement. A report of Austrian workers taking early retirement found a significantly raised risk of heart disease and death (although only among men)[29] and an English study found retirement dramatically increased the chance of being diagnosed with a chronic condition, severe cardiovascular disease and cancer.[30]

Not all studies report the same conclusions, however. A recent Chinese report found that health among white-collar male workers improved after retirement. An intriguing 2018 report using data from 19 European countries found that when one member of a household retired, their own health improved but that of their spouse declined as the spouse took less exercise, smoked more and drank more. Typically it was the wife whose health deteriorated (significantly) when her husband retired. There's a clear message to married/cohabiting women here that we don't think needs spelling out! (But just in case, we'll quote directly from the report: 'While female retirement has no impact on male health, male retirement has a significant negative effect on their wife's subjective health status.'[31])

Incidentally, a sharp increase in alcohol consumption is often cited in retirement studies,[32] as is depression and loneliness. But on the other hand, many find it easier to get more exercise and enjoy shedding the stress that work can bring. Disentangling retirement studies is complex. The data rarely tells us why people have retired (ill health? Compulsory?) or what they do after retirement. Often it's the transition that's explored, rather than the subsequent decades, which means we find out about those who died, but less about those who lived. The point is that shifting from full-time work to no work whatsoever is often traumatic. We think it's a model that needs changing. Consider Annabel's brother-in-law, a teacher. At 60, he downshifted from a full-time position to a part-time position. After a couple of years teaching part-time, he retired and began tutoring students from home. Not everyone has the opportunity to downshift their jobs in this way, and yet research shows that mid-lifers and older people benefit from working part-time (assuming they can afford it), using the extra free time for exercise, volunteering and hobbies that can keep them healthy. When researchers ran a series of cognitive tests on 6,500 older Australians they found that people over the age of 40 performed best when working 25 hours a week. Beyond that, 'fatigue and stress' took over.[33]

The issue therefore is not whether to work or not to work (although if the choice is that stark, Professor Maestas of Harvard Medical School has studied all the data and says the better option for ageing is to work[34]), but rather how to fill those retirement hours with purposeful, challenging and socially engaging activities.

For people who enjoy their work (such as SuperAger Douglas Matthews, on page 303), retirement holds few temptations. But for others (such as SuperAgers Helen Holder and Margaret Hibbert, on pages 302 and 307), retirement provided the opportunity to develop new careers and interests.

Retirement: we say

- Rewire, don't retire.
- If you enjoy your work, keep going.
- Alternatively, see if you can work part-time or on a project basis.
- If you don't enjoy your work, consider changing career. Many people successfully change career in their middle – and indeed their later – years (including one of the authors of this book and her mother).
- If your work isn't as enjoyable as you'd like but you'd rather not change jobs, try reframing. Instead of thinking of work negatively, reframe it as something that gives you purpose, provides camaraderie, pays you, and keeps your brain activated.
- Ask for a promotion or a different role.
- Discuss retirement with your partner well in advance and agree how you'll spend your newly leisured time.
- Think about using your leisure time for a combination of exercise, education, volunteering and other activities that extend both your mind and your network of friends.

Walk a dog

The health benefits of owning a dog are obvious: dogs need walking, caring for and a regular routine – all of which help us to age better. And then there's the sheer joy they bring into our lives. Who doesn't smile when greeted by an exuberant pooch? No wonder dogs are referred to as man's (and woman's) best friend.

Having a dog forces you out every day, whatever the weather. Research shows that walking a dog boosts physical activity among older people, especially during the winter.[35] Researchers found that owning, or walking, a dog was one of the best ways to beat the decline in activity that often happens in later life. Dog owners were moving 30 minutes more than non-dog owners per day, on average.

Even this small amount of exercise can have a huge impact on health: a study of more than 3 million Swedes aged 40 to 80 found that dog owners had a lower risk of death, due to cardiovascular disease or other causes, during a 12-year follow-up period.[36] There may be other factors: stroking a pet has been found to raise levels of oxytocin, known as the 'love hormone', and to lower levels of cortisol, the stress hormone.[37]

Dogs provide companionship, which might also improve their owner's health. The Swedish study found that single people benefited the most:

A very interesting finding was that dog ownership was especially prominent as a protective factor in persons living alone, which is a group reported previously to be at higher risk of cardiovascular disease and death than those living in a multi-person household. Perhaps a dog may stand in as an important family member in single households. The results showed that single dog owners had a 33 per cent reduction in risk of death, compared to single people without dogs.

An Australian study of over 5,000 people found that pet owners had lower blood pressure and cholesterol levels than non-pet owners, despite similar body mass index and socio-economic profiles.[38] The pet owners took significantly more exercise than those without pets.

Having a dog means that your home might not be, ahem, as clean as it could be – and that's a good thing. Dogs contribute to the microbiome of our homes, which helps build our immune systems. The *New York Times* recently asked, only slightly tongue in cheek, 'are pets the new probiotic?'[39] Dog ownership increases the quantity of 56 classes of bacterial species in the home.[40] It's possible that dog owners benefit from contact with this wider variety of microbes, which in turn increases the microbiota in our gut.

Harvard Medical School advises 'get healthy, get a dog',[41] explaining that in addition to the enforced exercise, dog ownership can:

- Help you to be calmer, more mindful, and more present in your life.
- Improve the lives of older individuals by providing companionship and a reason to exercise.
- Make you more social and less isolated.

Dog ownership: we say

- You don't have to own a dog to reap the health benefits of looking after one: schemes like Borrow My Doggie mean that you can walk a dog without having to own one.
- If you're concerned about training or owning an energetic puppy, consider adopting. Dog charities often find it hard to place older dogs, which typically need less exercise.

- Caring for a dog doesn't come cheap, there are food and vet bills to consider. Make sure you've assessed the costs first.
- Ownership is more responsibility at a time when you might feel overwhelmed and sandwiched between a growing family and elderly parents.
- We've found dog owning hugely social – from puppy training classes to dog walking with friends (and together as we wrote this book) to swapping dog tips with strangers.
- As mums of teenagers, we've found shared dog walks a good time to discuss more difficult subjects, away from screens and social media.

CHAPTER 9

Work That Brain

Three decades ago, neuroscientists noticed how those with the highest levels of education appeared to have the lowest rates of dementia. Things became more interesting when it was found, at autopsy, that some of these highly educated brains were in fact riddled with the plaques and tangles of Alzheimer's, and yet, in life, these people had displayed no signs of cognitive impairment.

The term 'cognitive reserve' was coined to explain this extraordinary capacity. Think of it as the difference between a car that's stumped by a road closure and simply stops – versus a car able to read a map and navigate around the road closure, via a different route.

The argument goes like this: if you've spent your life building and using your brain, it might be resilient enough to circumnavigate brain diseases such as Alzheimer's, Parkinson's and strokes. Research has since borne this out in countries with highly educated populations,[1] and many scientists now believe that building cognitive reserve can reduce our chances of neurodegenerative disease. Some experts believe that as many as 25 per cent of people with dementia are able to fully mask their symptoms – thanks to their cognitive reserves.

Although the majority of studies have correlated education levels and/or high career attainment with cognitive reserve (most recently in Japan[2]), a recent study in the *Journal of Gerontology*[3] suggests that many other factors can play a role, from card games and board games, to volunteering, to visiting art galleries. Therefore, if you don't have a PhD, don't worry. The most important thing is to keep your brain busy, curious and challenged.

Work your brain to build your cognitive reserve

Don't wait until it's too late. Building cognitive reserve is a life's work, starting in childhood, so start as soon as you can, by consciously exposing your brain to cognitively stimulating life experiences. If your job bores you, think about changing it. Sign up for that course you've always wanted to do. Spend time with people who make you think.

We're very partial to attending lectures, reading books (see 'Why Do Book Readers Live Longer?' on page 229), visiting galleries and museums (take the audio guide to keep you focused) and playing board games, not to mention watching TED talks and taking the odd course (we're fans of www. thegreatcourses.com).

- There's never been a better time to access lectures, talks and the great minds of the genuinely gifted. Swap your Facebook scrolling for a podcast, a YouTube seminar or a TED talk.

224 THE AGE-WELL PROJECT

- Sign up for a course and learn something new.
- Seek out new opportunities at work or volunteer for positions where you'll learn something new.
- Swap your annual pool holiday for a learning holiday. Lots of organisations offer a holiday that combines learning a new skill with rest and relaxation. Try www. GoLearnTo.com.

Do something creative

Being imaginative builds cognitive flexibility.

Question: What do the following have in common – Doris Lessing, Georgia O'Keeffe, Pablo Picasso, Louise Bourgeois, Sonia Delaunay, Barbara Cartland, Marc Chagall, Oscar Niemeyer and E.M. Forster?

Answer: They all lived well into their nineties and without succumbing to dementia. And – of course – they're all well-known writers and artists. But it's not only these well-known names that lived to a ripe old age. A look at the Wikipedia register of notable centenarians tells a similar story. Of 115 centenarians over the age of 102, 40 per cent were professional writers, artists or musicians. We'll call them 'artistic creatives' for want of a better term. A Wiki study might not be statistically robust, but this anecdotal research reflects other studies, including a report in the *Journal of Aging and Health*,[4] which found that people following creative vocations often live particularly long and active lives.

A recent study found that creative thinkers are more likely to engage disparate networks across the brain,[5] keeping their neurons firing. We also know that many artistic creatives work all their lives, never retiring. They are often (but by no means always) exceptionally self-disciplined, another character trait linked to longevity.[6] Our Wiki research bears this out: the second largest category of centenarians after artistic creatives were athletes and those from the military. We doubt there's much on the subject of self-discipline these people don't know.

Psychologists believe that artistic creatives often have a deep sense of purpose, but, more importantly, they have an openness to new ideas and a flexible attitude to change, something referred to as cognitive flexibility. Michelangelo famously said 'I'm still learning' at the age of 87. He lived for another two years. According to one study, a flexible mind is one of the most important ingredients in fending off cognitive decline among the elderly.[7]

Researchers believe that having cognitive flexibility means we react differently to stress, something found in many creatives, who tend to see new things as challenges or imaginative opportunities rather than threats. Consider Matisse who, when confined to a wheelchair and no longer able to paint, began working on his celebrated paper cut-outs.

Can, therefore, adopting a creative pastime give us the cognitive flexibility of an artist? Quite possibly. Doing something creative involves organising one's thoughts and feelings, opening up to new experiences, and learning to think imaginatively. In other words, learning to engage disparate neural networks. Studies suggest that creative expression also relieves stress and depression and could help those with arthritis, asthma, even cancer.[8] Imaginative writing has been found to reduce pain and stress and to strengthen the immune system.[9] Studies have linked dance and drama to improved cognition, and musical training to improved neural connectivity. The brain, it seems, relishes the imaginative challenge of making art.

Age is no impediment. You might not have had a typically creative career, but if you've always wanted to try sculpture, pottery, photography, acting, composing or writing poetry, find a course and have a go. Who knows, it might help develop your cognitive flexibility. At the very least, it will add to your social enrichment and your cognitive reserve – without a single side effect.

Develop your creativity: we say

- Try a creative holiday: plenty of companies now offer painting/writing/cooking (and so on) holidays while some schools and universities provide cost-effective courses when their students have vacated. In the UK we like Marlborough College Summer School, https://summerschool.co.uk/find-course.
- Find an evening or weekend class at a local art school or through your local council.
- Literary festivals often include inexpensive writing workshops. Find one near you.
- Take an online course, if you prefer. MOOC (Massive Open Online Courses) include free creative writing courses from some of the world's best universities: https://www.mooc-list.com/.
- Or just buy a sketch book, a paint-box, some clay, or a notebook – and have a go.

Embrace novelty: try something new

The brain loves novelty. When we experience new or different things, our brain builds new neural pathways. Sometimes called the 'novelty response', this reaction improves our memory and our ability to learn, and it can help us survive the threat of dementia. This is why experts suggest we constantly learn new things. Professor Michael Hornberger, Director of Ageing at Norwich Medical School and Head of Dementia Research at the University of East Anglia, urges us to seek novelty throughout our lives: 'Novelty is very important for the brain. The brain works harder when it's exposed to new things. Once we've learnt something it becomes a skill and the brain doesn't engage in the same way.'[10]

Blue Zones researchers confirm this. They claim that learning something new is one of the five scientifically proven ways of beating dementia: 'Knitting, playing board games or learning other crafts during mid-life can reduce memory loss by 40%–50%.'[11]

A study published in *Neuron* found that the parts of our brain known as the substantia nigra and ventral tegmental area (SN/VTA), which are closely linked to the hippocampus and the amygdala, and play large roles in learning and memory, are activated by new images, but only those that are positive (which is why we often recall holidays so clearly). Positive novelty enabled and increased the creation of new neurons, as well as rewarding the brain with a shot of dopamine. This was most marked when the stimulus was completely new. As researcher Dr Düzel explained: 'only completely new things cause strong activity in the midbrain area'.[12]

Coasting through a daily crossword puzzle is not enough.

Our brains, like our muscles, need stretching – and that means embracing novelty. Learning languages and instruments are invariably cited as the ultimate brain challengers, but we can stretch our brains in simpler and less intimidating ways. One of our favourites is regularly learning a new word, but visiting museums and galleries, grappling with a new app on your mobile phone or a new function on your laptop, trying out a new recipe, travelling and meeting new people, all help our brains to build new connections.

Conversely, researchers have found that watching TV is the activity least likely to build a healthy brain. According to Blue Zone researchers, elders watching TV for more than seven hours a day are 50 per cent more likely to experience memory loss.[13]

Now is the time to build novelty into your life. Try taking a new route to work or hanging new pictures in your house. Go somewhere new for a holiday. And when you get there, eat food you've not eaten before. Try a new exercise class. Choose a different genre of book to read. Cook from a new recipe. Learn a new craft or skill. Go on – challenge yourself. And when you've mastered it, find something else you've not done before.

Studies of SuperAgers suggest that exposure to novelty is one of the things these extraordinary people have in common, with travel and reading being two of their favourite pastimes.

Embracing novelty: we say

- Reading a book provides imaginative novelty, taking you to new worlds. Films and plays can do the same.
- Travel provides instant novelty, but it doesn't have to be

anything more time-consuming or expensive than walking a new route to work or exploring a corner of your city or county that you've not visited before.

- Local councils often provide a wide range of classes.
- Take every opportunity to meet new people.
- Try cooking a new dish once a week.
- Visit galleries and museums with changing exhibitions.
- Change your usual choice of music and try something different.
- Wherever and whatever, seek out novelty in your life.

Why do book readers live longer?

No research has *ever* linked staring at a screen with a healthy old age. Reading books, however, is an entirely different story. A Yale study of 3,635 over-fifties found that reading increased longevity by almost two years. As the researchers explained, 'Reading books provided a 23-month survival advantage ... The benefits of reading books include a longer life in which to read them.'[14]

A closer look at the study (in which other longevity factors, such as gender and education, were stripped out) shows that it's also *what* you read that counts. Readers of books out-lived both non-readers and readers of newspapers and magazines, while the researchers speculated that it was reading fiction that reaped the greatest benefits.

How long you read matters too. In the 12 years following the study, those who read for more than 3.5 hours a week were 23 per cent less likely to die, whereas those who read for less time were 17 per cent less likely to die. As the report authors said, those who read most lived longest, but 'as little as 30 minutes a day was still beneficial in terms of survival'.

In many ways, this is a baffling finding. After all, reading is sedentary and solitary, so what's going on? Can reading books really extend your life?

The authors identified two cognitive processes involved in book reading that could create a survival advantage. Firstly, reading books involves a 'slow, immersive process', a cognitive engagement in which we make imaginative connections, ask questions or absorb new vocabulary, for example.

Secondly, books 'promote empathy, social perception, and emotional intelligence', all processes that scientists now believe give us a greater chance of survival.

There are other reasons that might have escaped the authors but didn't escape my writer and reader friends. Reading books, particularly novels, alleviates stress by plunging us into a world other than our own. It can make us feel happy, engaged, grateful in a way that flicking through a magazine rarely does.

Reading can also help us sleep (almost every sleep expert advocates reading as a means of falling asleep). Scientists believe the process of reading replicates the eye movements we make during REM sleep, precisely the time we lay down memories.

Reading: we say

- Read in bed every night.
- Invest in books or visit your local library.

- Participate in a book club. Bookshops and libraries often have them or you can join an online book discussion group, like GoodReads.

Forget brain-training games

Should you 'brain train'? Will it prevent cognitive decline? The answer from us is a resounding no! We tried brain-training apps and games as part of our Age-Well Project, thinking, like many people, that they would keep our minds sharp. Instead we found ourselves compelled to keep playing in order to beat our scores. We also – to our horror – became tempted by the attractive, but expensive, in-app purchases (most brain-training games are designed to be addictive). After hours spent alone, hunched over screens, we felt no more mentally challenged than we had before. Incidentally, one popular American brain-training app was recently fined $2m for overstating its claims to improve cognition.

The latest research into brain training found that the skills learnt in one game did not translate to other, similar, cognitive tasks.[15] The trial investigated whether training on one memory task led to better performance on a similar task for which the participants hadn't been trained. It didn't. The participants became good at the one task they were trained for, but nothing more. The lead researcher concluded, 'If you're looking to improve your cognitive self, instead of playing a brain training test for an hour, go for a walk, go for a run, socialize with a friend. These are much better for you.'

Learn a language or an instrument

A healthy brain never loses the ability to learn and grow, a process known as plasticity. But we need to keep our brains plastic by adopting activities that force our brains to think, and therefore grow new neurons. The best way to grow these neurons, and build cognitive reserve, is not by doing the same things – such as sudoku and crosswords – over and over, but by challenging our brains to learn new things. In a marvellous TED talk, *Still Alice* author Lisa Genova says, 'You don't want to simply retrieve information you've already learned, because this is like travelling down old familiar streets … you want to pave new neural roads. Building an Alzheimer's-resistant brain means learning to speak Italian, meeting new friends, reading a book or listening to a great TED talk.'[16] Professor Hornberger confirmed this when we spoke to him, saying, 'it's no good doing a crossword puzzle every day. Try something new. Learning an instrument or language is particularly effective because of the complexity involved.'

Learn a language Being bilingual could delay the onset of Alzheimer's by four and a half years.[17] But you don't have to go that far: learning a new language has been shown to increase the size of the hippocampus, the area of the brain responsible for memory.[18] We've been learning French on and off for years, making use of the cheap, sociable classes run by our local council. A two-hour lesson feels like a brain workout!

Play a musical instrument Adults aged 60–83 who'd played an instrument for at least ten years scored better in non-verbal memory tests and executive processing than non-musicians.[19]

Your voice constitutes an instrument, so consider joining a choir. Professor Hornberger recommends singing, because not only does it challenge the brain, but it also offers social interaction (via a choir) while simultaneously providing a physical workout. We've tried singing lessons and – to our surprise – found that they worked our core muscles, improved our posture and made our brains ache from the effort of reading music. Perhaps just as importantly, singing made us feel supremely happy.

Bear in mind that the latest science suggests that doing a long block of study isn't the best way to learn. Learning in snatches – a little here and a little there – is not only more effective but can be fitted around a busy working day. And don't worry if you immediately forget what you've learnt. Scientists now believe forgetting plays a critical role in how we learn, forcing us to retrieve and re-engage with material which, in turn, deepens and extends our memories.[20]

Language and music: we say

- Seek out inexpensive language courses run by your local council or library service.
- Go online – thousands of tutors now offer inexpensive Skype language tuition.
- If your town has an overseas twin, make the most of it and get involved.
- Find a local linguist who can provide an hour of conversation over a coffee, or organise a conversation group for friends.

- Join a local choir. Many churches still have choirs, and if hymns aren't your thing, find your local rock choir at www. rockchoir.com.
- Worried you can't sing? Try www.tunelesschoir.com. It may have a choir near you.
- Learn an instrument.
- Join a local brass band, orchestra, quartet, jazz band. Or set one up.

Adopt a complex hobby or a challenging sport

If instruments and languages have little appeal, don't worry. The important thing is that your brain works to the point of aching. Hobbies and sports can work the brain muscles in exactly the same way.

Find a complex hobby: a study followed people who adopted a new hobby involving active learning and sustained activation of working memory (like digital photography or quilting, for example). The participants showed enhanced memory function after three months.[21] According to Professor Hornberger, 'anything new will be effective. It can be carpentry, crochet or knitting.'[22] Annabel studied photography before we started our Age-Well blog and her skills enabled us to grow the project, which resulted in this book. From small acorns . . .

Take up a new sport, or improve your skill at a sport you already enjoy: exercise is one of the best ways to keep your brain healthy. Cognitively challenging sports are even better, enabling the brain and body to be worked simultaneously. If the sport comes with a dash of social interaction, all the better. If you'd rather not take up something new, commit to dramatically improving your current sport.

Hobbies: we say

- Investigate classes at your local council.
- Inspire others with your experiences. We have friends who've taken up bell ringing, ceramics, upholstery and poetry writing.
- Dancing, tennis and ping-pong combine a brain and body workout (see Chapter 7) with social interaction.

Meditation

The busy-ness, stress and constant 'on' of modern life contribute to ageing, taking their toll both mentally and physically. Meditation can help reconnect with yourself and the world around you. When we started this project, we wondered how we could squeeze meditation into our lives. But meditation has proven highly effective, leaving us calmer and more clear-headed.

Meditation focuses on the breath, a mantra, or simply being present in our surroundings. Buddhists believe that it helps to relieve stress by enabling us to let go of the anxieties that contribute to inflammatory conditions. Research has shown that experienced meditators perceive less stress than non-meditators and have lower reactions to stress tests and lower cortisol levels.[23] Research conducted by the US Army also found that meditation reduces stress by stabilising the heartbeat.[24]

In one study, 20 people who'd been practising Zen meditation for at least an hour a day for at least 10 years were compared to 20 people who'd never meditated. The meditators had telomeres that were 10 per cent longer than those of the control group.[25] Dr Elissa Epel, whose work on telomeres is described on page 25, was one of a number of scientists who tested participants in a three-month, full-time meditation retreat in Colorado. She found that, at the end of the retreat, meditators had significantly higher telomerase activity than the control group.[26] 'If the increase in telomerase is sustained long enough,' Epel said, 'it's logical to infer that this group would develop more stable, and possibly longer, telomeres over time.'

If you're a beginner, fear not. Another study found that a mere 15 minutes a day of meditation increased the activity of the gene that makes telomerase, the enzyme responsible for extending telomeres. This short practice also enhanced the expression of genes associated with energy metabolism and mitochondrial function, while reducing the expression of genes linked to inflammation and stress.[27]

Meditation appears to have a powerful impact on the brain, leading to an increased ability to focus, and more positive emotions. Research suggests that the focus on breath has a direct impact on the brain by increasing levels of noradrenaline, a natural chemical messenger that helps the brain grow new connections.[28]

Meditation might also protect against age-related cognitive decline. A small study showed that regular practitioners of Zen meditation didn't lose grey matter in the brain or suffer reduced concentration when compared to a control group. The researchers said, 'These findings suggest that the regular practice of meditation may have neuroprotective effects and reduce the cognitive decline associated with normal ageing.'[29] A 2017 review of 13 other studies reached the same conclusion. The researchers said, 'Preliminary evidence suggests that meditation may offset grey matter atrophy.'[30] A very specific form of meditation, Kirtan Kriya, which involves chanting and finger movements, has been found to stabilise brain synapses and increase cerebral blood flow. A research team investigating its benefits concluded that it 'should be considered for inclusion as part of an Alzheimer's disease prevention programme, alongside other potentially beneficial modalities such as diet, exercise, mental stimulation, and social activity'.[31]

Meditation has also been found to promote empathy – something that benefits all humanity.

Meditation: we say

- You don't have to go on a three-month meditation retreat to feel the benefits. Try a mini-meditation: we have found that focusing on the breath or being aware of our surroundings for a few moments helps us feel calmer.
- Since discovering she has the ApoE4 gene, Susan does Kirtan Kriya every day. It's simple, quick and can be learnt from guides on YouTube. Chanting out loud might feel silly, but the evidence that it reduces Alzheimer's risk is compelling.

- We're always looking for ways to be active, but meditation can be very sedentary. Try a yoga class that incorporates both movement and meditation.
- There are some effective meditation apps: check out 'Headspace', 'Calm' and 'Insight Timer'. Look out for running and walking meditations, which mean you move as you meditate.
- Try a group class to enjoy the positivity and connection that comes from meditating with others.

CHAPTER 10

Have a Positive
Attitude to Ageing

How do you feel about getting older? If you're reading this book, you probably want to age as happily and healthily as possible. But how do you *really* feel about the thinning hair, sagging skin, creaking bones and inevitable decline that comes with age?

Negative stereotypes of ageing abound. If you believe the headlines, older people are bed-blocking, house-hogging drains on society. Researchers from University College London, asked participants in a longitudinal study about their perception of age discrimination. One-third said they'd experienced age discrimination. The figure was even higher for the over-sixty-fives.[1] No wonder it's easy to feel negative about growing old and the impaired health, loneliness and frailty that age can bring.

Thinking like this threatens our health, however. An Irish study found that older people with a negative attitude to ageing had slower walking speeds and worse cognitive abilities than those with more positive attitudes. This led study author,

Professor Rose Anne Kenny, to quip, 'The saying "You're as young as you feel" is true.'[2]

It's also true for long-term health. A British study, which followed 400 people aged 50 plus, for 18 years, found that those with a positive view of ageing had better functional health at the end of the research period. Once again, the better your attitude to ageing, the better your experience of ageing is likely to be.[3]

Unsurprisingly, negativity puts stress on the body. Older adults' levels of cortisol, a stress hormone, were tested over a four-year period. Their self-esteem was evaluated at the same time. The researchers found that when self-esteem decreased, cortisol levels rose, and vice versa. This association was particularly strong for people with a history of stress or depression.[4] Long-term elevated cortisol levels can impact heart health, sleep quality, weight and cognition.

We started our Age-Well Project because we didn't want to age like our forebears. Learning about healthy ageing has been tremendously empowering. We feel much more optimistic now that we understand how to manage our health in the years to come.

Cultivate the right attitude to ageing: we say

- Remember, you can control how you age.
- Arm yourself with knowledge, not just about your health, but about all your options as you age.
- Think about your finances. Where will you live? How much do you need to live on? Will you continue to work?

- Exercise: it reduces stress, increases life expectancy, reduces the risk of chronic illness and releases endorphins (the happy hormones).
- Explore self-help books and podcasts.
- Practise mindfulness, meditation, t'ai chi, qi gong or yoga.
- Volunteer in a sector that interests you.
- Find people who share your interests: join local groups and clubs.

Find your sense of purpose

When we interviewed nonagenarians for this book, we quickly became aware that all of them shared one particular trait: a deep sense of purpose.

In a study involving 6,000 people over 14 years and published in *Psychological Science*, Professor Nicholas Turiano came to the conclusion that having a sense of purpose reduced mortality risk.[5] This reflected several earlier studies that found a correlation between a sense of purpose and healthy longevity.[6] Doctor Robert Butler, founder of the International Longevity Centre, led an 11-year study that explored this correlation and found that those who had clear goals or purpose lived longer and with less disease than those who didn't. A later study of 136,000 Japanese and Americans linked a strong sense of purpose with a lower risk of heart problems.[7]

According to Blue Zone researchers, knowing your sense of purpose (they call it the 'why I wake up in the morning'; Dr Sara Gottfried, author of *Younger*, calls it simply 'the *why*'; and the

Japanese have a special word for it: *ikigai*) is worth up to seven years of extra life expectancy and is linked to a reduced risk of Alzheimer's, stroke and arthritis.

This may be because a sense of direction has been shown to have a positive epigenetic effect, switching certain genes on and off in a way that supports anti-inflammatory processes.

But having a sense of direction isn't the prerogative of the religious, or the ambitious, or even the artists we wrote about in Chapter 9. Anyone, whatever their circumstances and however menial their days might feel, can develop a sense of purpose. When the janitor at NASA was asked by President Kennedy what he did each day, instead of saying 'I sweep the floor', he famously replied, 'Mr President, I'm helping put a man on the moon.'

Unsure what your sense of purpose is? Try writing it down. Pay special attention to your reasons for wanting to age well. This will help you to stick to any lifestyle changes you make after reading this book. If you're unsure where to start, here are ours:

Annabel 'To walk the world's most beautiful wildernesses; to keep thinking, reading, writing and supporting the causes that matter most to me – for as long as possible.'

Susan 'To avoid getting dementia; to minimise any burden on my children; to keep my husband healthy; to spread the message that we can all improve how we age.'

And here's one we love from Maya Angelou 'My mission in life is not merely to survive, but to thrive; and to do so with some passion, some compassion, some humour, and some style.'

If you're still unsure, volunteering can help provide a genuine sense of direction. According to Blue Zone researchers, people who volunteer also have lower rates of cancer, heart disease and depression.

A sense of purpose: we say

- Put your purpose in writing and stick it on your fridge door (or anywhere you'll see it regularly).
- Consider volunteering.
- Re-train for a role with a greater sense of purpose.

Be grateful

Gratitude is one of the hottest areas of neuroscience. Not only is it hot, but it's also the simplest, easiest activity in this book.

Numerous reports suggest that grateful people experience fewer aches and pains, are happier and less depressed, sleep better, have lower blood pressure and better cholesterol.[8] Amy Morin wrote in *Forbes* magazine, 'being thankful throughout the year could have tremendous benefits on your quality of life. In fact, gratitude may be one of the most overlooked tools that we all have access to every day'.[9]

More recently, a brain-scanning study reported in *NeuroImage* suggested that making one's gratitude tangible (writing it in a journal or a letter, for example) has results that endure for months afterwards. The same study found that the more you practise gratitude, the more attuned you are to it and the more you enjoy its benefits.[10] Neuroscientist Dr Christian Jarrett suggests we think of our brain 'as having a sort of gratitude muscle that can be exercised and strengthened'. Apparently, using our 'gratitude brain muscle' causes a cascade effect, in which others are then able to feel more grateful and so receive the ensuing physical and emotional benefits too.[11]

A series of studies using brain MRIs found that the part of the brain known as the hypothalamus (which regulates a range of bodily functions, from our metabolism to hunger, growth and sleep) is activated when we think grateful thoughts or do something altruistic. Scientists don't yet understand why this happens, but it's not inconceivable that one day poor sleepers might be encouraged by their doctor to undertake gratitude exercises rather than pop a pill.

Another report found that people who feel grateful recover more quickly from trauma, while, according to Harvard Medical School, 'most of the studies published ... support an association between gratitude and an individual's well-being'. Research carried out by Professor Robert Emmons at the University of California found that people doing a daily gratitude exercise reported higher levels of enthusiasm, alertness and energy. Who doesn't want some of that?[12]

We regularly practise gratitude in our households, often expressing 'gratitude before meals', a sort of modern-day prayer for the faithless. It felt awkward at first, inevitably. But now it feels entirely natural and boosts the mood of all involved, while encouraging us to appreciate the many good things we have.

Gratitude: we say

- Remind yourself of the things you're grateful for.
- Lodge it in your brain by saying it aloud or writing it down.
- Share your gratitude with others.
- Make it a habit.
- Having trouble sleeping? Forget counting sheep, and play the Gratitude A–Z game instead: for each letter of the alphabet find something to be grateful for.
- You can also play Gratitude A–Z with children on long car journeys.

Develop your grit

SuperAgers is the term used to describe the very healthy elderly. We all know one or two: they're the ninety-year-olds doing press-ups in the park or the centenarian granny with a razor-sharp memory. Indeed, we interviewed several for this book, and you'll find them on pages 302–11.

One of their defining features, according to Professor Lisa Feldman Barrett, is their grit: the personal and cognitive resilience that enables them to bounce back from setbacks and adapt to negative or difficult circumstances. Feldman Barrett has studied SuperAgers and describes this as 'the ability to use your unpleasant feelings as fuel ... as a signal to keep going'. Instead of avoiding the difficulties and hardships of life or letting them overwhelm us, we must learn to see them as obstacles to be faced and overcome. Feldman Barrett prefaces this by explaining that most middle age people opt for easier lives, shying away from things that are difficult and challenging. But this isn't what we should be doing. To keep our brains wired, she recommends we 'engage in strenuous mental activity on a regular basis, enough to make you feel unpleasant in the moment ... and dive into it until your brain hurts'. This means finding something genuinely intimidating and having a go (like learning Mandarin or the violin). She urges us to adopt the same approach with exercise – making it vigorous and pushing ourselves 'past the point of unpleasantness'.[13]

Neurologist Professor Emily Rogalski has also studied SuperAgers. She found them to have a unique personality profile including high levels of resilience (grit), optimism and perseverance. This reflects a growing body of evidence finding higher levels of resilience in the long-lived.[14] The Blue Zoners from Sardinia, Ikaria (Greece) and Nicoya (Costa Rica) make it clear in interviews that the hardship they've endured required mental stamina and strength – personality traits that the American National Institute on Aging also found to be common in those over the age of 95.

Research into resilience has consistently found those with greater grit to have an 'internal locus of control', a belief that *they*, rather than their circumstances, are in control of their lives. And yet psychologists believe anyone can develop grit.[15] Where, then, do we start?

Developing grit: we say

- Get enough sleep – it's easier to be positive when you're well-rested.

- Make exercise and eating well a priority – it's more difficult to have grit if you're frail or unwell.
- Know your purpose (see 'Find Your Sense of Purpose' on page 241).
- Celebrate successes, however small.
- Have a wide circle of supportive friends and nurture those friendships.
- Re-frame adversity as a challenge rather than as a threat.
- Develop a positive attitude (as discussed at the beginning of this chapter).

Laughter: the best medicine

It's a cliché and sounds a little trite, but could laughter really help us to live better and longer? We were sceptical. But our investigations revealed enough solid science to make it plausible. And now we're doing our very best to laugh more.

Studies have linked laughter to better immunity, improved mood, reduced stress and even improvements in rheumatoid arthritis. A study from Oxford University found that laughter releases endorphins, which dull pain.[16] Leeds University found that a good laugh helped a sample of 337 people with leg ulcers to heal more quickly.[17] Laughing, the author explained, gets the diaphragm moving, which propels blood round the body. A study from Vanderbilt University in America found that laughing helped people lose weight. Those who laughed for 15 minutes a day lost an additional 2kg over a year.[18] A study from Loma Linda University discovered that laughter lowered stress hormones and enhanced immunity, not only while the respondent was laughing but for 24 hours afterwards. Moreover, these effects started with the *anticipation* of a good laugh. Simply expecting to laugh, it appears, is enough to trigger the process of stress reduction and immunity boosting.[19]

The University of Maryland Medical Center speculated that laughing could reduce the risk of heart disease, reflecting a Japanese study involving 21,000 people (aged 65+), which found that non-laughers had a 21 per cent higher risk of heart disease and a 60 per cent greater risk of stroke when compared to those who laughed every day.[20] Another Japanese study found that laughter reduced the pro-inflammatory cytokines in rheumatoid arthritis that cause the joints to swell and become stiff and painful.[21] Further studies suggest that laughing affects cognition and recall. If we find something funny, we're more likely to remember it. A recent meta-analysis identified laughter as having 'significant positive effects' on the well-being of adults over the age of 60.[22]

Meanwhile, laughter therapy and laughter yoga programmes have been associated with lower blood pressure and reduced depression. One study found laughter yoga to be as effective as therapy for elderly women with depression.[23]

It's not only laughter that benefits us. A smile might be all it takes. Researchers at America's Wayne State University studied photographs of smiling baseball players and found that bigger smiles correlated with longer life (seven years of extra life to be precise). 'Smile intensity,' the author explained, 'correlated with marriage stability and satisfaction.'[24]

No one really understands why the body responds so favourably to smiling and laughter, but it seems that when we laugh, a wave of electricity washes over our cerebral cortex, the outer layer of our brain, which activates immune cells, reduces stress hormones like cortisol, and releases feel-good endorphins. Moreover, our muscles relax, we breathe in lungfuls of oxygen and our blood flows more freely (rather like a mini workout). When we smile, our brains release dopamine, which makes us feel good.

Laughter (of the right sort, of course) is a highly effective way of bonding. Professor Robert Provine, an American neuroscientist, spent ten years studying laughter and came to the conclusion that laughter is inextricably linked with socialisation, arguing that 'the health benefits may be coincidental, consequences of its primary goal – bringing people together'.[25]

Either way, we decided it was time to get more laughter into our lives.

Laughter: we say

- Fake it – the brain doesn't know the difference between a fake smile and a real one. It only recognises the muscle movements in your face. Smile and you might actually feel happier, regardless of how cheesy your grin.
- Watch funny films. Keep a collection of films that make you laugh.
- There are hundreds of hugely talented comedians – try watching their shows, live, on TV or YouTube.
- Read funny books (humour is very subjective, but we're partial to Richmal Crompton's Just William series, Helen Fielding's Bridget Jones novels and James Hamilton-Paterson's Gerald Samper trilogy).

- Follow funny people on social media. An amusing tweet or Facebook post might be all it takes to liven your day.
- Visit comedy clubs.
- Try laughter yoga.
- Play funny games.
- Spend time with people who make you smile, laugh and/or think, and steer clear of doom-mongers, energy sappers and human irritants.
- Explore the App Store. We have it on good authority that there are several genuinely funny apps out there.
- Pin these words from the poet e.e. cummings on your office wall or on your kitchen fridge: 'The most wasted of all days is one without laughter.'

CORNERSTONE FOUR

Creating The Right Environment For Good Sleep, Lustrous Looks and Enhanced Health

Our sleep patterns change as we age. Sleep, for those over the age of 50, often becomes more erratic with less rapid-eye movement (REM) sleep, and more frequent periods of wakefulness. And yet it is at this time of life that we desperately need quality sleep.

Over the last few years multiple studies have linked poor sleep to Alzheimer's disease, cancer, obesity, depression, diabetes, heart attacks, strokes, poor memory and a shorter life in general.[1] We've also learnt that good sleep means a healthy microbiome, happy telomeres, improved immunity and better skin.

More recently, however, studies have suggested that too much sleep is as detrimental to our long-term health as too little sleep.

Much of this research has been written up in rather terrifying books – something entirely unconducive to a good night's sleep.[2] *All you need to know is that a stretch of deep sleep will help your long-term health. As Professor Hornberger explained to us, 'it's not about the amount of sleep but the quality of sleep. Constant interruptions to our slow-wave sleep can contribute to protein accumulation in the brain.'*

In the following chapter we consider the many factors that help us get a good night of shut-eye and we explain how to engineer your own sleep hygiene programme ('sleep hygiene' is the new term for having the right factors in place to help you sleep better).

In this section we also review several other factors affecting our ability to age well, from looking after our teeth, eyes, skin, hair and immunity to choosing supplements and avoiding pesticides, pollution and medications that may be detrimental to our health. We believe – as do many of the experts we spoke to – that the next big threat to our health and to the health of our planet is pollution. By nourishing our bodies and challenging our brains, we can build our defences against pollution. But is this enough? If you live in a polluted area, consider avoiding arterial roads, filling your homes with the right houseplants and using an air purifier. The most important contribution we can make, however, is to play our part in reducing global pollution: drive less, consume less, recycle, shop locally, lobby for improved regulation. Sadly, this is a subject beyond the scope of this book. But we urge you to read more (we cover as much as we can on our website) and do what you can.

CHAPTER 11

How to Sleep

Like many others, we've battled with insomnia over the years. But by reading and researching, and a process of trial and error, we've radically improved our sleep, both in duration and in quality. First, we had to grasp how much sleep was enough.

How much sleep is enough?

Sleep experts routinely suggest that we should aim for at least seven hours of sleep a night. We're all different, so you might need more. A few people function competently on less. But most researchers have concluded that – for the bulk of us – seven to eight hours is the sweet spot. A recent study found that, from a sample of 12,775 people aged 30–74, those who slept seven hours a night had the healthiest hearts.[1]

A review of the sleep habits of more than 1.3 million people showed that the risk of death increased by 12 per cent for those who slept for less than six hours a night, and by a rather staggering 30 per cent for those who slept more than nine hours.[2]

Ignore headlines suggesting that one night of poor sleep will kill you. Recent research has overturned the studies (and misappropriated headlines) that threatened imminent death for those of us not getting seven hours of quality sleep every night.[3] A report from Flinders University in Australia found absolutely no connection between occasional sleeplessness and mortality.[4]

Another study, from Stockholm University, looked at the sleep habits and health of 43,000 people and found that it was the average amount of sleep over time that mattered. In other words, on the odd occasion when you've had a sleepless working week, a weekend lie-in is an effective means of catching up. The same report linked less than five hours and more than eight hours' nightly sleep with higher rates of mortality, consistent with previous studies.[5]

Remember, however, that we have genetic predispositions to sleep. If your parents and grandparents slept for longer-than-usual, you might simply need more sleep than others.

Regular hours are the secret to sleeping well

As mothers of young children we dreamt of having a lie-in (which never happened). Now we're mothers of teenagers we look on with envy/frustration as they emerge from their beds at midday. But we've learnt that the long lie-ins we once craved aren't good for us as we age. It's all down to our circadian rhythms.

Almost every animal on the planet, from fruit flies to humans, has a circadian rhythm regulated by its genes. In humans, this 24-hour rhythm controls virtually every process in the body including our sleep–wake cycle, metabolism and brain function.

Our circadian rhythms naturally change as we age, which is why we often wake earlier in the morning. Scientists have discovered that our bodies develop a whole new set of genes in later life, which affect these rhythms: essentially, our body clock gets out of sync. Researchers analysed brain tissue from people who had died either before the age of 40 or over the age of 60. The younger brains had, as the researchers expected, 'classic' body clocks. But the older brains revealed disrupted 'classic' body clocks and an additional new set of body clock genes.[6] The researchers believe that the body creates these genes in an attempt to protect the nervous system from the ageing process.

If getting older disrupts our circadian rhythms anyway, then disturbing our sleep patterns still further with sporadic late nights and lie-ins isn't going to help. Research done on mice reveals that a disrupted body clock causes faster ageing.[7]

Getting up at the same time each day 'anchors' our circadian rhythms and gives them a cue for when we should be awake. From that point, we go through our day becoming increasingly alert, and then increasingly tired, as time passes. If we disrupt this pattern by having a lie-in, it's harder to get to sleep in the evening. So a Sunday lie-in, however appealing, will make getting to sleep on Sunday night more difficult.

Your sleep routine: we say

- Go to bed! It sounds so ridiculously simple, but in our time-poor lives it's all-too-easy to watch another episode on Netflix/put on a wash/reply to emails. Meanwhile, sleep gets pushed back later, becoming ever more elusive.

- Go to bed at the same time each night.
- If you're finding it hard, try setting two alarms each day: one for the morning and one for the evening. Set the evening alarm to remind you to start winding down for bed.
- Allow an hour of winding down time before bed. Most sleep experts recommend reading a book as the best preparation for sleep.

Why you need to know about blue light

For people living in 1900, mass production of the electric light bulb was world-changing. The planet was, literally, a brighter place. Once-dark evenings now gleamed with harsh electric light. Roll forward a century, and our lives are illuminated by a constant electric glow: not just from light fittings, but from televisions, phones, alarm clocks and screens.

Our bodies aren't designed to deal with all this artificial light. Our delicate circadian rhythms are programmed to respond to daylight, not the round-the-clock gleam of electronic devices. The knock-on effect is devastating: when our bodies are exposed to more light, they produce less melatonin, the vital sleep-inducing hormone. No wonder there's a global pandemic of sleeplessness.

Not all light is created equal. Basic physics: light is made up of the seven colours of the rainbow. Different coloured light has a different impact on our bodies. In the daytime, we need blue light to boost mood, alertness and reaction times. But that's exactly what we don't want at night. The screens we're glued to in the evenings emit blue light, and keep us awake. Meanwhile, some of the energy-saving LED light bulbs we're encouraged to buy emit more blue light, so it's increasingly hard to avoid it in our homes. Researchers at Harvard compared sleep patterns of people exposed to regular room light before bed, to those of people exposed only to dim light. Unsurprisingly, the volunteers who spent their evenings in brightly lit rooms produced melatonin later in the evening, and only half as much as the people who spent their evenings in gloom.[8]

Harvard researchers also tested the effects of exposure to blue light, against exposure to green light. The blue light suppressed melatonin production for twice as long as green light, and shifted circadian rhythms by three hours as opposed to one and a half hours.[9] Red light has the least impact on melatonin production, so if you need a night light, make it a red one. Research from Israel showed that looking at a screen emitting red light between 9pm and 11pm had almost no impact on melatonin production.[10] The team also conducted a relatively simple experiment. Participants spent an evening away from all forms of artificial light. The next day they were tested to see how well they had slept and how well they functioned. They then spent evenings in front of light-emitting screens and were tested again. Guess what? Their sleep quality wasn't as good, nor did they function or concentrate as well the next day.[11]

Light-emitting screens: we say

- Create your own electronic 'sundown': turn off all screens an hour before bed, and dim the lights.
- Keep all devices out of the bedroom. Buy a cheap old-fashioned alarm clock so that there's no excuse to keep your phone in the bedroom.
- Wear blue-light blocking glasses if you have to look at screens in the evening. Everything looks a bit sepia, but it does work. Amazon has a range of reasonably priced ones.
- Download a free app like f.lux, Twilight or Redshift onto your computer. These programmes can be set to reflect sunrise and sunset wherever you are, so that your screen emits less blue light in the evenings.
- Experiment with night-shift settings on your phone so that there's less glare.
- If you use a Kindle or other e-reader, turn any back lighting right down and use the front lighting. That way the light is aimed at the text, not your eyes. Research shows it takes longer to nod off when using a back-lit e-reader.

Creating the right sleep environment

Not everything works for everyone, and sleep problems are rarely solved (ahem) overnight, but let's start with the basics.

Keep the bedroom dark and quiet Remove anything likely to beep, whirr, squeak (or snore?) and invest in blackout blinds *and* curtains. We both live under a flight path, and overcoming the noise pollution has taken time and experimentation. Annabel sleeps with earplugs or an audio book (find a narrator with a low soothing voice and a plot you already know, without musical interludes). Friends of ours swear by white noise (a consistent, single-frequency sound like the whirring of an overhead fan) and/or pink noise (a combination of sounds of varying frequencies such as wind in the trees) apps. According to one study, pink noise reduces brain-wave complexity and induces better quality sleep.[12]

Keep the bedroom cool We never turn on the heating in our bedrooms except on the iciest of winter nights. Use a hot water bottle or an electric blanket to warm your bed if need be. Today's electric blankets offer a range of temperature settings and automatic shut-offs. Creating the right level of warmth was critical in our search for a good night's sleep. On which note, we urge you to experiment with nightwear and bed socks. Mid-life plays havoc with female body heat, and sleep experts agree that temperature is critical (most suggest keeping the bedroom at 16–18°C).

Have the right kit Make sure you're sleeping on a supportive mattress (these should be changed every 20 years and regularly turned), with decent pillows (treat yourself to the very best you can afford and change them every few years). According to sleep expert Dr Neil Stanley, quality pillows are vital for keeping the neck and spine aligned as we sleep. Have the right weight of duvet to prevent waking from being either too cold or too hot.

Keep the window or door fractionally open This reduces the amount of carbon dioxide in the air and has been shown to improve sleep quality.

Scent your bedroom with chamomile, lavender, vetiver or a sleep blend, using an oil diffuser, an hour before you go to bed. Anecdotal evidence suggests that it helps soothe frazzled nerves. If it has no other effect, at least your room will smell drowsily delicious.

Experiment with how you sleep Sleeping on one's side has been linked to reduced risk of Alzheimer's and Parkinson's by researchers who used MRI scans to investigate the sleep and health of rats (not people). The brains were more effectively cleaned of 'waste' – the amyloid and tau plaques and proteins thought to build up and lead to Alzheimer's and Parkinson's diseases – when the rats slept on their sides rather than their backs or fronts.[13] However, later research suggests that sleeping on one's back is the best for avoiding aches, pains and heartburn. We say comfort is key.

Getting to sleep

When it comes to falling asleep, we're all different. We need to understand what's preventing us from falling asleep and we need to experiment as we search for a cure. If it's not the kit (lumpy mattress, over-thick duvet, pyjama buttons in the wrong place, and so on), is it the evening tipple or the laptop in bed? Where falling asleep is impeded by physical pain or extreme stress (like bereavement), or where the following day necessitates some sleep, a sleeping pill might be the best option. Otherwise throw out the pills, start a sleep journal and prepare to experiment.

Avoid stimulants in the evening Be wary of consuming stimulants in the eight hours before you sleep – that includes alcohol, caffeine and anything containing nicotine. We keep our evening drinks to a single glass of wine, unless we're celebrating. If you've had your genome done you'll know whether you're a fast or slow metaboliser of caffeine – take a cue from your genes.

Exercise in the evening A recent study found that evening exercise increased deep sleep, unless it was extremely vigorous and done within an hour of sleep-time.[14] New research links a lack of deep (slow-wave) sleep to the higher levels of tau implicated in Alzheimer's disease and cognitive decline.[15]

Avoid overstimulation during the evenings If you know that a late, boozy dinner hinders your sleep, decide which you'd rather have – the fun night out or the good night's sleep – and either turn down the invite or factor a nap into the following day.

Allow time to unwind Meditation, reading, listening to music or having a warm bath can help. We try not to schedule difficult conversations, watch distressing TV, open post, check email or social media during the hour before bed. Most sleep experts advise reading from something non-thrilling. We've found short stories, recipe books and poetry to be particularly effective.

Avoid blue light and screens Decide what time you'll turn off the house wi-fi or collect in the gadgets and devices (10pm in our homes). And stick to it. See the previous section on 'Why You Need to Know About Blue Light'.

Don't take meds (or supplements) before bed Some medications and supplements interfere with sleep. Try to take them earlier in the day, if possible.

Staying asleep

Once asleep, we'd all like to stay asleep. Research suggests that nights of broken sleep can be as ageing as not sleeping enough. A 2012 study published in the *Journal of the American Geriatrics Society* showed that older women with repeatedly broken sleep were three times more likely to go into a nursing home than the women who slept the best.[16] These are our top tips for staying asleep:

Exercise during the day If you're physically tired you've more chance of staying asleep. Research consistently links exercise to good sleep. The more you exercise (and the greater the vigour), the better you sleep. A study published in the *Journal of the American Medical Association* found that people who exercised regularly slept almost an hour longer each night and fell asleep in half the time it took others. A report from America's National Sleep Foundation found that any exercise improved sleep, but that vigorous exercisers reported the best sleep – and this is certainly what we've found.[17]

Expose yourself to natural light every morning We spend at least 30 minutes outside, either dog walking or cycling to work, every morning without fail (it's one of the benefits of having a dog, see page 218). Sleep experts have found morning sunlight to be critical for re-setting circadian rhythms, thereby enabling good night-time sleep.

Take an afternoon walk somewhere green and leafy Researchers found that an afternoon walk among trees adds an average of one hour's additional sleep compared with those either not walking or taking an urban walk.[18]

Eat the right food in the evening (see Chapter 1), not too late and not too much of it. Again, both sleep experts and longevity experts recommend not eating a large meal within three hours of sleeping.

But don't go to bed hungry Sleeping on an empty stomach isn't ideal, and a new study (although very small) posits that 30g of cottage cheese an hour before bed might actually be beneficial to our health, helping us to repair muscle and boost immunity as we sleep.[19]

Reduce evening liquids If you're waking to go repeatedly to the bathroom and not managing to return to sleep, try switching the bulk of your daily fluids to the morning and not drinking much liquid after 6pm.

Keep a pen and paper by your bed If you wake with something on your mind, write it down (in the dark) and promise to deal with it in the morning.

Don't lie awake worrying If you can't get back to sleep, get up. Annabel wrote a first draft of a novel in the early hours of the morning. Other friends of ours do yoga or housework. Take comfort from the history and theory of biphasic sleep, which suggests that we were never designed for a single eight-hour stretch of sleep. Historic accounts show our ancestors socialising, walking and working in the middle of the night, while those in hot climates often split their sleep between night-time hours and an afternoon siesta.

See your GP, if you've had sustained insomnia for several weeks. But avoid sleeping pills except in an emergency. We've not come across a single sleep expert who advocates routinely taking sleeping pills.

Sleep: we say

- Aim for seven to eight hours of sleep each night, unless you're genetically predisposed to need more or less.
- Exercise during the day, in natural light.
- Don't be afraid to exercise in the evening: a new study suggests evening exercise may increase length of *deep* sleep.
- Keep regular hours.
- Avoid blue light and screens before bed.
- Make sure your mattress, pillows and bed linen aren't keeping you awake.
- Keep your bedroom at a coolish temperature that works for you.

- Keep your bedroom dark and quiet, and experiment with sleep-inducing oils.
- Try sleeping in a different position.
- Use steady, consistent white or pink noise and/or earplugs to blot out external sounds.
- Allow time to unwind before bed.
- Can't sleep? Don't fret – get up and do something.

Food for better sleep

Changing our evening eating habits was pivotal in addressing our poor sleep. We changed not only what we ate but when and how much we ate.

The key to sleep, as we have seen, is melatonin, a hormone that declines as we grow older. Melatonin, as it happens, is also a hormone that promotes longevity – so there are many reasons to include it in your diet. A few foods contain melatonin naturally (cherries and oats, for example), whereas vitamin B_6 makes melatonin. As so few foods contain melatonin, we focused on increasing B_6 in our evening meals. Good sources include sunflower seeds, pistachio nuts, tuna and wild salmon, avocado, chicken, cooked spinach, bananas and prunes.

The amino acid tryptophan also helps to produce melatonin and is found in fish, nuts and seeds, eggs, soya beans, bananas, whole grains and dairy. Magnesium is another nutrient vital for sleep (found in almonds, leafy greens, bananas and fish), as is calcium (leafy greens, yoghurt and cheese). Some of these ingredients contain a double whammy of sleep-inducing nutrients.

Prunes, for example, contain B_6, calcium and magnesium, bananas contain B_6, magnesium and tryptophan, oats contain B_6 and melatonin, and pistachio nuts contain B_6 and magnesium. The perfect evening meal for a good night's sleep is quite possibly banana porridge with prunes and pistachio nuts – something most of us would associate with breakfast.

Complex carbohydrates are also important, not only because they make one feel full (and who wants to go to bed feeling hungry?) but also because they help the brain absorb tryptophan. Sweet potato is often cited by nutritionists as good starchy sleep food, because it does all this and includes B_6, calcium and magnesium. As a bonus, sweet potatoes also include fibre to keep you feeling replete as you sleep.

We also identified foods to avoid in our evening meal: aubergines, tomatoes, pineapple, chocolate, fermented/cured foods and wine all contain tyramine, a brain stimulant. Therefore, we waved bye-bye to one of our favourite suppers: moussaka with a large glass of wine followed by a chocolatey pudding. From then on, supper was invariably eggs or fish, leafy greens and a whole-grain carbohydrate, followed by a banana and a handful of cherries or perhaps yoghurt with prunes. Very spicy, heavy, fried and sugary meals have also been linked to poor sleep.

Perhaps our most peculiar experiment was with kiwi fruit. Research from Taiwan's Taipei Medical University found that volunteers eating two kiwi fruit before bed for four weeks fell asleep more quickly, slept more deeply and for longer. It's not a study that we'd normally pay much attention to. But the medic and science writer Dr Michael Mosley also trialled the use of kiwi fruit on an insomniac shift worker in a BBC TV programme – with good results. As kiwis are inexpensive and ubiquitous (not to mention rich in antioxidants, serotonin, fibre and vitamin C), we saw no reason not to eat a couple every night. After two weeks of kiwis-before-bed, in tandem with less alcohol, the sleep-friendly foods above and some daily exercise, we noticed an immediate improvement to our sleep. But was it really the kiwi fruit? We'll never know, but studies say the placebo effect is easy, cheap and ... remarkably effective.

Meanwhile we're sticking (mostly) to the 23 sleep-friendly foods recommended by sleep expert Dr Michael Breus:[20] beef, tuna, salmon, halibut, pumpkin, asparagus, beetroot, artichokes, seaweed, avocados, leafy greens, broccoli, beans, almonds and walnuts, oats, buckwheat, Greek yoghurt, low-fat cottage cheese, bananas, cherries, kiwi, lavender or chamomile tea.

Food and sleep: we say

- Eat foods that contain, or help to produce, melatonin.
- Eat foods rich in calcium, magnesium and vitamin B_6, such as those listed above.
- Include complex carbohydrates.
- Avoid foods that stimulate.
- If all else fails, try a kiwi fruit.

Should we take a nap?

Now, we know napping doesn't suit everyone, but we're firmly of the belief that poor sleepers (that's us) need naps, if only to catch up on lost sleep. But is napping good for us? And do nappers live longer or less diseased lives?

Apparently so. In a study of 3,000 older Chinese, researchers found that intermediate nappers (those sleeping for less than 90 minutes) had less cognitive decline than non-nappers or long nappers (over 90 minutes).[21] Lab-based experiments reflect this, finding napping improves cognition and lowers blood pressure.[22]

Another Chinese study found that those napping five to seven days a week had sustained attention, better non-verbal reasoning ability and improved spatial memory, with those sleeping for between 30 and 60 minutes performing best. In this study habitual nappers were also found to sleep better at night, countering some experts who believe napping disrupts night-time sleep.[23] Other studies have found that naps restore all the biomarkers affected by disrupted sleep, thus reversing the damage accrued by successive nights of insomnia. One small study even found that a 30-minute nap could relieve stress and bolster immunity as well as reversing the hormonal impact of a poor night's sleep.[24]

It gets better: researchers from the University of Pennsylvania found that a nap improved thinking and memory skills, making the brain perform as if it were five years younger. A study from the Sorbonne University in Paris found that naps lowered stress and boosted immunity. A study from NASA found that pilots and astronauts had a 45 per cent improvement in performance and a 100 per cent improvement in alertness after a 40-minute nap. A study from Germany found that 'strategic nappers' experienced a five-fold improvement in retrieving information from memory. Other studies have found that: the creative side of the brain is highly active during napping (artists everywhere, take note); that napping, when combined with moderate exercise, improves night-time sleep quality; that naps can lower blood pressure when taken after doing something stressful; that naps improve tolerance and reduce frustration (parents of young children and teenagers, take note).

Matthew Walker is a sleep expert and author of *Why We Sleep: The New Science of Why We Sleep and Dream*. When it comes to ageing, he's crystal clear: not enough sleep means a shorter lifespan. But for people with regularly disrupted sleep, napping can redeem their health and potentially restore their lifespan.

Walker cites a study involving 23,000 Greek men who, forced to give up siestas over a six-year period, increased their mortality rate by 60 per cent. Heart disease risk rose the most. On the Blue Zone Greek island of Ikaria, however, naps are still part of the culture: its men are four times as likely as American men to reach the age of 90. Coincidence?

While most research errs on the positive side of napping, extended naps (over 90 minutes) can be detrimental, and some research suggests napping isn't good for everyone. Indeed, some of Walker's own studies found that napping did not always compensate for disrupted sleep. We, however, never turn down the opportunity for a nap, particularly if we have a long night ahead of us. If Winston Churchill, Bill Clinton and Richard Branson managed a daily power nap, why shouldn't you?

Naps: we say

- Napping can be carried out anywhere free of interruption: a car, a sofa, even a floor. Turn your phone off and close your eyes.
- Don't nap too late in the afternoon or you might find yourself unable to sleep later.

- It's a myth that older people need less sleep – indeed they're more likely to have disrupted sleep and so are more likely to benefit from a nap. If you've had a bad night, take a nap.
- Remember, the sweet spot appears to be 30–40 minutes of shut-eye. Set your alarm if need be.

CHAPTER 12

Looking and Feeling Good

The state of our health is invariably reflected in how we look and feel. While sound sleep plays a crucial role so do other factors in our personal environment. To look and feel our best (peachy skin, healthy looking hair, strong teeth, clear eyes, a robust immune system capable of fending off common viruses) we need to examine other elements of how we live. Not only do we need the right food, but we need pesticide-free food, clean and unpolluted air, medication that doesn't harm us, sunlight in the right dosage and (possibly) the right supplements taken in the right way.

Skin

Our skin is our shield: the biggest and busiest organ of our bodies, protecting us from pain, temperature fluctuations and the elements. As we age, our skin loses collagen (the main structural protein in our connective tissue) and becomes less elastic.

It's more fragile and susceptible to trauma, and it is easier to cut and bruise. Nor does it heal as well. For women, loss of collagen is linked to the decline in oestrogen that comes with the menopause. This drop in oestrogen also causes bone density loss. A study of menopausal women by Yale School of Medicine found that those with the deepest wrinkles and the least elastic skin had the lowest bone density.[1]

This makes sense: both bones and skin are made of collagen. Our bones are highly mineralised but still 50 per cent collagen. Beauty really is more than skin deep. Similarly, both bone and skin are broken down by free radicals.

The simplest way to avoid free-radical damage to the skin is to stop smoking and avoid sun. We use a high factor sunscreen on our faces in the summer, and get the vitamin D we need by exposing our arms and legs to the sun.

We've long known about the damage to our skin from sun and cigarette smoke. But dermatologists are now exploring a new threat: pollution. Polluted air, particularly in urban areas, contains toxic particles including particulate matter (PM) and nitrogen dioxide (NO_2). Research suggests that these increase skin ageing, with NO_2 specifically responsible for an increase in age spots.[2] Professor Krutmann, who led the research, said: 'UV [damage from the sun] was really the topic in skin protection for the last 20–30 years. Now I think air pollution has the potential to keep us busy for the next few decades.'

There are two proven ways to protect our skin from the ravages of modern living: quality sleep and a good diet. A study comparing women who slept for five hours a night with those who slept for seven to nine hours found that the skin of good sleepers recovered better after exposure to ultraviolet light.[3] How we eat is also critical: junk food and sugar wreak havoc with our complexions. Excessive consumption of fructose – the sweetener found in many processed foods – accelerates ageing by damaging collagen.[4]

Research published in the *International Journal of Cosmetic Science* showed that post-menopausal women given a cocktail of isoflavones, lycopene, vitamin C, vitamin E and omega-3 had a marked reduction in their wrinkles after 14 weeks. Isoflavones are the phyto-oestrogens found in beans (particularly soya), lycopene is found in watermelon and cooked/dried tomatoes, vitamin C in oranges, vitamin E in avocados and omega-3s in nuts and oily fish.

Foods for healthy skin: we say

Get plenty of these foods:

- Deeply coloured fruits and vegetables – add them to every meal. Mix berries into your porridge (frozen are fine). Chop colourful vegetables such as sweet potatoes, aubergine and red pepper into small cubes, toss them in olive oil and seasoning, and roast in a hot oven for 40mins. Use in everything, and top with a poached egg for a simple supper.
- Chia – we love these little seeds, which swell up when soaked in water or milk. They're packed with omega-3, an essential fatty acid that helps nourish the skin.
- Soya – we avoid over-processed soya milk, but love edamame beans. Most big supermarkets sell them frozen and podded. We add them to salads and soups because

research shows that soya might help heal some of the sun's photo-ageing damage.

- Millet: proof that not all superfoods are expensive, this gluten-free grain, traditionally fed to cattle and birds, is packed with the collagen-forming amino acids methionine and lysine. We use it instead of rice or pasta.
- Dark chocolate: everyone's favourite superfood. Cocoa contains high levels of flavanols, which protect the skin from sun damage and make it look smoother.

In addition:

- Wear a good-quality sunscreen in the sun, ideally without benzophenones, which are currently being investigated for their role in hormonal interference. You don't need pore-blocking factor 50 sunblock to sit in an office all day.
- Ignore the glossy marketing campaigns of global beauty brands. Moisturise regularly, use a serum and seek out products with fewer chemicals (avoiding phthalates and parabens for example, which researchers think might disrupt hormones). The easiest way to do this is to invest in certified organic skincare brands.
- Try an inexpensive jade or rose quartz skin roller. Used by Asian women for centuries, they soothe, smooth and de-puff the skin, helping it absorb moisturiser.
- As we age, our faces lose volume and our face muscles lose tone. Facial exercises can help strengthen the muscles

of the face. Try the exercises in *The Ultimate Facercise* by
Carole Maggio.

- Foundation protects the skin from pollution. Find an anti-
pollution serum and use under a foundation with an SPF
for extra protection.

Hang on to your hair

There's something deeply upsetting about losing your hair. And
yet hair loss is increasingly common as we age. Many factors
contribute to hair thinning and shedding, in addition to ageing:
male-pattern baldness, androgenic alopecia, menopause, poly-
cystic ovarian syndrome, lupus, thyroid problems and psoriasis,
for example. Hormonal change can wreak havoc, as can medications such as the contraceptive pill, antidepressants, anti-ulcer
drugs and beta blockers. Certain hairstyles can aggravate hair
loss too. In a review of 19 studies, researchers at Johns Hopkins
University found a 'strong association' between certain scalp-
pulling hairstyles and the development of traction alopecia,
gradual hair loss caused by damage to the follicle from prolonged
tension on the hair root.[5]

Studies have linked hair loss to deficiencies of vitamin D
and iron,[6] as well as to very low-protein diets. When Annabel's
hair began falling out in handfuls, she overhauled what she ate,
adding protein-rich foods such as fish, eggs and liver, making sure
she had a good source of protein at every meal. She researched
the best foods for hair and stuck the list on her fridge: salmon,
walnuts, almonds, sweet potato and carrots, leafy greens, lentils,

sunflower seeds, Brussels sprouts, blueberries, Greek yoghurt, oats, bananas, beef, poultry, oysters, eggs and soya beans. These foods contain a mixture of the most important nutrients for hair: protein, iron, biotin, zinc, vitamins C, D and B, silica (a trace mineral essential for hair), and an amino acid called lysine.

Hair is a slow responder. While poor diet or stress can show up in skin within weeks, it can take months for your hair to reveal quite how unhappy it is – either by coming out in great tufts or by becoming weak and brittle. The reverse is true too. After 12–18 months of a Mediterranean diet with extra protein, Annabel's hair began to grow again.

It wasn't exclusively the result of diet. She also changed how she treated her hair. Chemicals can damage and weaken hair, as can heat. She started colouring only her roots and stopped using a hair-dryer. She stopped combing her hair when it was wet, but most significantly of all, she stopped conditioning her hair after shampooing, switching to conditioning beforehand instead. While conditioning first probably has no effect on generating new hair, it makes hair look fuller. When hair is lank and thin, conditioner clings to it making it look even lanker and thinner.

Shampoos claiming to reverse hair loss are best avoided, according to Sally-Ann Tarver, trichologist at The Cotswold Trichology Centre: 'Hair loss shampoos do not promote hair growth, whatever they may contain.' It's more important to avoid using shampoos containing sulfates (research suggests sulfates can damage hair cuticles) and conditioning or pearlising agents, which are designed to make the hair glossy but actually leave a film which clogs follicles and hinders new hair growth.

Hair loss: we say

- Visit your GP if your hair loss is serious.
- Change your diet to include good sources of protein and plenty of vegetables and nuts.
- Look for a sulfate-free shampoo without silicones, conditioning or pearlising agents.
- Review how you treat your hair, cutting down on restrictive styling, blow drying, combing-while-wet and over-dying.
- Try the condition-before-shampooing technique.
- Check with your doctor or pharmacist if you think your medications might be affecting your hair.
- Protect your hair from prolonged sun exposure by wearing a hat.

The science of vitamin supplements

The debate over vitamin supplements has never raged as loudly or vociferously than at present, so what are we to make of it?

A review of all the data and single randomised control trials published between 2012 and 2017 found that multivitamins, vitamin D, vitamin C and calcium (the most commonly taken supplements) showed no advantage in the prevention of cardiovascular disease, heart attack, stroke or premature death. 'We were surprised to find so few positive effects of the most common supplements,' explained the lead researcher. 'So far, no research has shown us anything better than healthy servings of less-processed plant foods including vegetables, fruits and nuts.'[7]

In fact, the study did find a very small advantage to supplementation with folic acid, either alone or combined with B vitamins.[8] At the other end of the scale, niacin and antioxidant supplementation 'might signify an increased risk of death'. In other words, taking supplements might actually be detrimental to our health. This reflects earlier reports linking beta-carotene supplements with an increase in lung cancer, stroke, heart disease and a shorter life span,[9] and a recent report linking synthetic vitamin E with a greater risk of prostate cancer.

The tide appears to be turning against vitamin supplements. More and more reports suggest that most supplements have limited effects while some may do more harm than good. It seems that supplements are only needed when a good diet can't be followed or vitamin deficiencies have been professionally diagnosed. This was the view of every expert we interviewed for this book.

What about the ever-popular omega-3s? It's a not dissimilar story: an analysis of 20 studies found that those taking omega-3 supplements didn't lower their risk of heart disease, stroke or death,[10] although a later report found high doses of omega-3 via supplements helped people who already had cardiovascular disease.[11] Nor did omega-3 supplements prevent cognitive decline in older people, despite earlier studies suggesting that heavy fish eaters were less likely to develop dementia.[12]

And probiotics? Research suggests that probiotic supplements are also unreliable, with a new study suggesting that probiotic supplementation might even be dangerous. A small study found that excessive probiotics could cause brain fog, bloating and wind when they lead to bacterial growth not only in the colon but in the small intestine. The study author urged probiotics to be viewed as a drug rather than a supplement.[13] Another new study suggests that probiotics might be harmful to anyone with a compromised digestive system and that there's no one-size-fits-all probiotic supplement.[14]

One of the intrinsic problems of supplements is knowing exactly what's in them, and whether the elusive ingredient has survived the manufacturing and transportation process. More than almost anything else, we purchase a supplement on trust alone.

The other reason supplements might not work is because food appears to act synergistically in our extraordinarily complex bodies. No one understands exactly how, but phytonutrients appear to work in partnership not only with each other but with vitamins, minerals, bacteria and even fibre, altering biochemicals in our gut and blood. Most of the experts we interviewed said that the secret of a good diet lay in the *interaction* of nutrients, the inter-relationship of bioactives, vitamins, minerals, probiotics and prebiotics, rather than in a single ingredient: 'Just because a goji berry has been tested positively in a petri dish doesn't mean it has the same effects in a human body, and the same goes for a supplement.'[15] And: 'Nutrients in food interact favourably with each other and synergize. We need to focus on foods.'[16]

Our research suggests that there are three supplements worth taking: vitamin D, if you don't have access to regular sunlight; zinc, if you're succumbing to a cold; and folic acid if you're pregnant or wanting to conceive.

Several studies have linked vitamin D to longer life[17] and we examine these in our section on vitamin D. As our subject is longevity, we'll leave out the folic acid explanation. Supplementation with zinc, unlike vitamin C, has repeatedly been found to shorten a cold and reduce the severity of symptoms.[18]

There's an argument for taking a multivitamin as we age:

our bodies change at middle age and older people, for example, don't absorb as much B_{12} from their diet. Taking a multivitamin could be an insurance strategy that also stops us worrying. As Professor John Mathers, director of the Human Nutrition Research Centre at Newcastle University, said: 'It won't do any harm so if it makes you feel better, why not?'[19]

Supplements: we say

- Don't waste money on supplements (except vitamin D and zinc in certain circumstances) unless your diet is compromised.
- If you think you're nutrient-deficient, ask your GP for a blood test.
- Resolve any deficiencies with diet as well as a supplement.
- Eat lean meat occasionally to prevent iron and B_{12} deficiency.
- If you're elderly and taking a multivitamin, make it iron-free. Research has linked excess iron in the brain to Alzheimer's in some people.[20]

Susan's supplements

Susan takes three supplements. She often works on location, leaving her reliant on catered or commercially produced food. Supplements are an insurance policy for her, particularly as she's inherited a copy of the ApoE4 gene.

Co-enzyme Q_{10} is an antioxidant, generated in the liver through a complex, multi-step process and found in mitochondria, the 'batteries' of our cells, where it aids energy production. The latest theories about the origins of Alzheimer's disease point to disruption of the mitochondria, which supply energy to the brain, by beta-amyloid. Research shows that pre-treating mito-chondria with a variation of CoQ_{10} before they are exposed to beta-amyloid has a protective effect.[21]

Cells lacking CoQ_{10} are less efficient: replenishing CoQ_{10} when levels are low can reverse insulin resistance.[22] However, researchers believe that oral CoQ_{10} supplements might not effec-tively restore mitochondrial CoQ_{10} due to low absorption rates. It's possible to buy 'body ready' supplements of the active ingre-dient in CoQ_{10}, ubiquinol, so that's what Susan takes, although they are more expensive.

Vitamin B The B group of vitamins is another substance that the body finds increasingly hard to absorb as we age. Over the age of 50, gastric acid secretion diminishes, making it harder for our bodies to extract B vitamins (particularly B_{12}) from animal products. Susan takes a supplement two to three times a week, not daily. There are several reasons she wants to make sure she has enough vitamin B:

1   She lives and works on busy roads. A small study has shown that vitamin B can mitigate the effects of pollu-tion on the cardiovascular system.[23]
2   Folic acid (another member of the B group of vitamins) has been shown to reduce stroke risk.
3   She rarely eats meat and wants sufficient B_{12}. Vitamin B_{12} is found in soil, absorbed by animals as they graze and passed on through meat. Our ancestors routinely consumed vegetables fresh from, and tainted by, the

earth. But, these days, our vegetables arrive mud-free – and therefore B_{12}-free.

Vitamin D – the key to healthy ageing?

No other vitamin has been quite as applauded, or inspired such controversy, as vitamin D. Wading through the recommendations on when to take it or how much to take (not to mention whether you should bother taking it) is baffling, to say the least.

Over the last decade research has linked vitamin D deficiency (something the World Health Organization believes has now reached 'an international epidemic of frightening proportions') with a wide range of diseases, from cancer to Alzheimer's, from respiratory infections to multiple sclerosis, from heart disease to rickets, from rheumatoid arthritis to diabetes and colon cancer. The days of vitamin D being considered beneficial for nothing but bones are long gone.

Vitamin D is made primarily from sunlight on our skin. Most medics agree that those of us who live in the northern hemisphere (or with our bodies covered) do not get enough. In addition, as we age, our skin is less able to convert sunlight to vitamin D. Few foods contain much vitamin D (oily fish, dairy, pork, eggs, mushrooms, cheese and fortified cereals contain varying amounts), so for these reasons some governments now offer free supplementation to the elderly.

More recently, very early stage research from the Buck Institute for Research on Aging suggests that vitamin D might suppress a significant pathology of ageing – making it a critical supplement for longevity. This would explain why those living in less sunny areas appear more prone to some of the diseases we associate with ageing. The researchers found that vitamin D extended median lifespan by 33 per cent in nematode worms, slowing the age-related mis-folding of hundreds of proteins and prompting Professor Lithgow at the Buck to say:

> vitamin D_3 ... suppressed protein insolubility in the worm and prevented the toxicity caused by human beta-amyloid which is associated with Alzheimer's disease. Given that aging processes are thought to be similar between the worm and mammals, including humans, it makes sense that the action of vitamin D would be conserved across species as well.

He speculates that people with vitamin D deficiencies might age faster.[24]

After reading hundreds of reports on the dangers of vitamin D deficiencies, we felt compelled to take a supplement throughout winter and early spring. If you work long hours indoors, year-round, we suggest supplementing throughout the year.

How much should you take? Again, medics disagree. Of course, the right level of supplementation should be determined by how much vitamin D we already have, how much we obtain from our diet, how readily our skin and/or gut absorbs it and so forth. For this reason, we recommend getting yourself tested (ideally in winter and summer). If that's not possible, take a tip from the experts.

The good news is that many of those who've studied the effects of vitamin D are (more or less) in agreement. Professor Steve Jones (who spent two years studying the effects of sunlight on humans) takes 1,000 IU in winter and spring. Professor Janice Schwartz, who studied vitamin D supplementation in the elderly, recommends 800–1,000 IU daily. Boston University vitamin D expert Dr Michael Holick also recommends 1–2,000 IU a

day – unless you're getting plenty of sun exposure. And Professor
Graeme Close at John Moores Liverpool University advises elite
athletes to take 2,000 IU and takes the same himself; however,
some vitamin D researchers take 5,000 IU daily (and more) and
this is the recommendation of the Vitamin D Council.

If you've had your genotype tested, look for a negative variant
of the vitamin D receptor gene (VDR), which allows your cells
to effectively absorb vitamin D. If you have a weak variant, you
might want to take the advice of Dr Sara Gottfried and 'raise
your intake of vitamin D beyond the standard recommendation
of 1,000–2,000 IU per day'.[25]

Although there's little evidence of vitamin D supplementation
being harmful at these levels, we should draw your attention
to growing speculation that vitamin D supplementation might
interfere with the delicate machinations of the microbiome.[26]
Very large doses (above 10,000 IU) have side effects that include
constipation and kidney damage.

Vitamin D: we say

- Get your vitamin D serum levels tested. Researchers
  don't agree on a minimum healthy level, but our research
  suggests that for optimal levels it should be at least 30
  nanograms per millilitre (30ng/ml or 75nmol/L) and ideally
  above 50ng/ml (125nmol/L).[27]
- Supplement with 1,000 IU of vitamin D_3 during months of
  low-angled light (that's winter and spring in the UK), and
  continue year-round if you can't get outdoors. Raise or
  reduce this according to your blood serum levels.

- Eat a diet rich in vitamin D (wild salmon is one of the very best sources, but a tin of sardines typically provides 100 per cent of your RDA).
- Get sunlight on your skin whenever you can – which means exposing arms, face and neck (or equivalent) without sunscreen for 15–20 minutes, depending on your location, every two days.

Look after your teeth

For years we paid scant attention to our bleeding gums. As sleep-deprived working mothers we wanted to fall into bed as quickly as possible. Nightly flossing was a step too far, while morning flossing was simply inconceivable. For years we brushed as quickly as possible, while small wailing children hung from our legs and a day of meetings and presentations beckoned. And as for regular visits to the dentist, suffice to say we organised them for our parents and children, but at the cost of our own teeth. Family and work took precedence in those days.

Looking after your teeth and gums, however, might be one of the smartest things you can do to age well. Indeed, those of us with a full set of teeth at the age of 74 are significantly more likely to make it to 100. Meanwhile, those of us that have lost five or more teeth by the age of 65 have a much greater risk of ending our days prematurely, with diabetes, heart disease and osteoporosis.[28]

Our mouths are home to more than 700 species of bacteria, which hide and multiply beneath our gums where regular brushing can't reach. From here they spread to other tissues via the bloodstream, where they can do untold damage, even helping to create environments in which cancer cells can take root.

Experts now believe that gum disease might be a trigger for pancreatic cancer as well as heart disease and diabetes. It's been linked to dementia, obesity and even poor sleep, and several gerontologists list flossing – either with floss or interdental brushes, although the latter are now thought to be more effective than floss – as one of their top tips for healthy ageing.

It was the words of Professor Eberhard, Chair of Lifespan Oral Health at the University of Sydney, that really struck home for us. Poor oral hygiene, he explained, effectively undoes any age-defying physical exercise, because, while exercise strengthens and extends our telomeres (see Chapter 1), gum disease weakens and shortens them. His words filled us with horror: all our hard work exercising was being undone by failing to floss.

A study from the University of Buffalo involving 57,000 women over seven years found that those with periodontal disease or inflamed gums had a 46 per cent higher risk of death from any cause. Study author, Professor LaMonte, said, 'Oral screening in midlife may be just as important as screening for cholesterol, high blood pressure or glucose tolerance.'[29]

Meanwhile, other experts suggest that unchecked gum disease could lead to impaired cognition. The West Virginia University School of Dentistry found that people with tooth and gum disease scored lower on memory and cognition tests, while Columbia University found that older Americans with the most inflamed gums were up to three times more likely to have poorer memory and cognition.[30] A large study from Taiwan found that people with ten years of chronic gum disease were 70 per cent more likely to develop Alzheimer's.[31]

The good news? Gum disease can easily be reversed by following expert tips for maintaining scrupulous gum health:

- Use an electric toothbrush with revs of at least 4,000 and keep it fully charged. Brush properly, following the instructions.
- Brush for 2 minutes twice a day.
- Use a daily interdental toothbrush (or floss if the spaces between your teeth aren't wide enough for a brush).
- See your hygienist and dentist every six months.
- Don't waste money on mouthwash, special brush heads or other gadgets claiming to clean between teeth.

Eyes

We dread the thought of losing our sight; not being able to see our children's faces or read a favourite book seems too cruel. Age-related macular degeneration (AMD) is the leading cause of blindness in the developed world. Every day in the UK 200 people develop the condition. Other eye conditions, including glaucoma, cataracts and sight-related diabetic complications, are increasingly common in countries with an ageing population.

AMD damages the macula, the small spot near the centre of the retina needed for sharp, central vision. The macula allows us to see objects that are straight ahead. Sufferers of AMD are left with peripheral vision, or, in extreme cases, no vision at all. Age is the most obvious risk factor for this debilitating condition: most sufferers are over 60, although symptoms can start after 50. Other risk factors include smoking, family history, high blood pressure, dehydration, being overweight and high levels of saturated fat.[32]

Numerous studies have pointed researchers in the same direction: the best way to protect our eyes from AMD is to avoid smoking, keep active and eat healthily.[33] Our eyes need specific carotenoids (a type of plant-based antioxidant) called lutein and zeaxanthin. These two macular pigments effectively operate like a pair of in-built sunglasses, protecting plants from too much sun. They do the same for us by protecting our corneas from excessive blue light.[34]

To get this protection we need to eat plants rich in macular pigments. Nature makes them easy to spot: anything bright yellow, orange or green is a rich source. Corn (maize) is the richest plant source: more than 85 per cent of the total carotenoids are lutein and zeaxanthin. Orange peppers, kiwi fruit, grapes, spinach, oranges, courgettes, and different kinds of squash are all great sources.[35] Green leafy veg such as kale are rich in lutein but not zeaxanthin. Surprisingly, carrots contain almost no lutein or zeaxanthin. They're packed with another carotenoid, beta-carotene, which the body converts to vitamin A to support eye health. It won't make you see in the dark though!

Damage to the retina doesn't just come from the sun: electronic screens emit blue light too. Continuous exposure eventually leads to the death of light-sensitive photoreceptor cells in our eyes. These photo-receptor cells need molecules called retinal to sense light. Recent research has found that when retinal molecules are exposed to blue light they create toxins that kill off photoreceptor cells.[36] It goes without saying that we need to limit screen time, particularly in the dark, to protect our eyes.

In the same way that we need to have our blood pressure, cholesterol and bone density checked as we age, so we should have regular eye tests. Ask your optician for a full retinal picture and a deep tissue scan of your optic nerve. This will enable her to identify any underlying issues such as thinning of the peripheral vision or detaching of the retina. Even if you have no problems now, the tests will give a baseline for future comparison. Our optician recommends a full eye scan every two years from the age of 50.

Protecting your eyesight: we say

- Get your eyes tested regularly: our eyesight changes rapidly from the age of 40. Wearing the wrong glasses could cause eye strain.
- Wear good-quality sunglasses on sunny days – even in winter. The sun might feel weaker in winter, but because it's low in the sky it can damage the eye.
- Eat orange, green and yellow foods every day.
- The omega-3s in vegetable oils, such as olive oil and argan oil, might help keep eye cell membranes flexible.[37]
- Exercise improves circulation, which in turn improves the amount of oxygen sent to the eyes, promoting the elimination of toxins for better eye health.
- Take regular screen breaks to rest your eyes. Close your eyes or – even better – take a walk and look at the view.
- Make sure you've got good light to read by. Invest in reading lamps if you need to.
- Wear safety goggles for any form of DIY or crafts involving chemicals or sprays.

Colds, cancer and a healthy immune system

Since we started the Age-Well Project the number of colds we succumb to each year has decreased dramatically. A strong immune system is critical as we age, for two reasons:

1   Our immune systems fight whatever comes their way, from colds to cancer. Scientists describe cancer as 'a failure of the immune system'.[38]
2   The immune system's response to colds triggers more inflammation in the body. Inflammation is at the root of much of the ageing process.

Our immune system functions by sending out white blood cells to destroy any antigen it detects. An antigen could be a virus, like a cold, or bacteria. It could also be a dead or faulty cell from our own body. It's these faulty cells that have the potential to become cancerous, but the immune system is designed to hold them in check. When our cells divide (as they are programmed to do) tumour-suppressor enzymes check them over to make sure that the cell's DNA has been replicated correctly. When there are too many errors, the enzymes ensure the cell kills itself in a process called apoptosis. If a cancer cell survives this, white blood cells – lymphocytes – seek out and destroy them. Therefore, the stronger the immune system, the better the response.

The system fails when cancer cells 'trick' the immune system into thinking that they are, in fact, healthy cells. Cancer manipulates the immune system by sending signals to the immune cells to switch off.[39] Some cancers have the ability to 'hide in plain sight', using the immune system to mask their presence.

Cutting-edge research focuses on teaching the immune system to recognise cancers and destroy them.[40]

It's generally thought that the immune system weakens as we age, making us more prone to everything from colds to cancer; however, research indicates that, as we age, the immune system actually *over*reacts when confronted with a virus, which in turn creates inflammation in the body.[41] The lead researcher of one study explained, 'It is possible that heightened immune responses—rather than defective immunity—attack the body and lead to disease.' This inflammation makes us sicker when we pick up a cold, thereby speeding up the ageing process.

A strong immune system relies on a healthy microbiome. Seventy per cent of the immune system is located in the gut. It needs good bacteria to perform its work – so that means plenty of probiotics and prebiotics and very limited antibiotics. The immune system and good bacteria in the gut work together to fine tune the body's response to invaders and keep the immune system in balance.[42] Gut bacteria help the immune system's T cells to develop, essentially 'teaching' them to tell the difference between a foreign substance and the body's own tissues. When this system becomes unbalanced, autoimmune diseases such as psoriasis, Crohn's and rheumatoid arthritis can develop.[43]

Supporting your immunity: we say

- Eat dark leafy greens, lettuce, cabbage, broccoli, Brussels sprouts, carrots, tomatoes, onions, garlic, mushrooms, berries and seeds – particularly pomegranate seeds.

- Shiitake mushrooms have a powerful effect on the immune system – sauté and eat them on toast for a quick weekend breakfast or add to a stir-fry. If you've got a cold, try a simple miso soup with mushrooms, ginger and greens.

- Research on vitamin C supplementation isn't conclusive, but there seems to be consensus on zinc. A daily dose of 10mg while you're under the weather reduces the duration and symptoms of a cold.[44]

- Elderberry extract has also been found to reduce the severity and duration of colds.[45] Find a brand fortified with zinc.

- There's no need to feed a cold: let your body rest and heal. Reduce your food intake, focus on fruits and vegetables – especially greens – either raw or in soups.

CHAPTER 13

How the Environment Impacts Ageing

Few of us give a second thought to the air we breathe, but is this sensible? A recent State of Global Air[1] report suggests that 95 per cent of the world's population breathes excessively polluted air, resulting in over 6 million premature deaths a year and making pollution the fourth deadliest health risk after smoking, poor diet and high blood pressure. Meanwhile, a *Lancet* commission went further, blaming pollution for 9 million premature deaths a year.[2]

A growing body of evidence also suggests that air pollution might have more of an impact on how we age than previously thought. We know that inhaling air pollution – a generic term for the cocktail of nitrogen dioxide, polycyclic aromatic hydrocarbons (PAHs), and particulate matter (PM) – increases our risk of lung cancer, heart disease, strokes and asthma. But new studies suggest it could also be linked to dementia, high blood pressure and diabetes.

Researchers at the University of California found that women living in areas with raised exposure to PM2.5 (these are the particles so small they can slip through the finest of filters) had twice the dementia risk, particularly those carrying the ApoE4 gene.[3] A study of 6.6 million Canadians found that those living within 50 metres of a major road were 7 per cent more likely to develop dementia than people living over 300 metres away, where PM levels were up to ten times lower.[4] A review of studies, analysed in *Neurotoxicology* and including countries as diverse as Taiwan, Sweden, China, Germany, the US and the UK, found the same association between pollution and dementia in every country but one. Meanwhile, both studies of mice and MRI scans on human brains also attest to a possible link between air pollution and cognitive impairment,[5] while a large Chinese study found that exposure to air pollution damaged intelligence, particularly in the elderly and particularly in men.[6]

When television presenter and medic Dr Xand van Tulleken was tested after a few minutes exposed to vehicle emissions in a typical city street, he found PM had lodged in his lungs and passed into his bloodstream, that his blood pressure had risen and his arteries had constricted, reflecting studies linking air pollution with hypertension and diabetes.[7] A new study in the *European Heart Journal* links air pollution to more than 2 million deaths a year from heart disease,[8] while a recent study of rats found inflammation and cancer-related genes in the rats exposed to long-term pollution.[9]

Professor John Mathers of Newcastle University considers pollution to be 'the next potential threat to our health'. He told us that pollution damages cells, resulting in inflammation. More optimistically, he believes an anti-inflammatory diet might help to mitigate the effects of pollution.

We live on arterial roads that reverberate, day and night, with lorries, buses and cars, while a succession of aeroplanes rumbles overhead. In other words, our families are subject to constant pollution. Like most people, we can't simply move house.

It's not entirely out of our control, however. Our research suggests that there are simple things everyone can do, while we press for governments to take action, with the first and foremost being to switch to a Mediterranean-style diet. A diet rich in antioxidants (that means fruit and vegetables) appears to provide some protection against the ravages of pollution.[10] Meanwhile, we've filled our homes with pollution-absorbing plants, following research from NASA that identified the 50 best plants for removing chemicals from the air. We've also invested in air purifiers: advances in technology mean that air purifiers are more effective than ever before.

Minimising pollution: we say

- We try our hardest not to drive our cars. The fewer of us that drive, the better our quality of air. Besides, air pollution is always worse *inside* a vehicle.
- When walking and cycling, choose back streets over arterial roads and keep as far away from slow-moving traffic as you can.
- Every decision you make impacts air pollution: buy local; choose less packaging; re-use and recycle.
- Hedges reduce pollution and capture PM on their leaves: consider planting an evergreen hedge in front of your house.

- Continue to open your windows regularly – internal air can be just as bad.
- Fill your house with greenery to absorb chemicals. Research from NASA suggests red-edged dracaena and peace lilies are particularly effective.
- Invest in an air purifier and rotate it around your house.

You can explore the data at www.stateofglobalair.org. We're keen campaigners for cleaner air and would urge you to join us. There are several charities doing valuable work in this area.

The possible effects of pesticides

Several scientists have speculated about the correlation between the rise of degenerative disease and pesticide usage. Of course, correlation doesn't mean causation. But could there be a link? Would we be better avoiding exposure to pesticides as part of our project to Age Well? And how should we do this?

As we wrote this book, the first individual to sue for damages, after a history of long-term exposure to a commonly used pesticide led to terminal cancer, won $289 million in compensation. Thousands of cases are now pending and we're watching with (horrified) concern. Much of the pesticide debate centres on the widespread use of glyphosate, the active ingredient of most weed killers used worldwide in farming, park maintenance and gardening. Traces of glyphosate, described by the World Health Organization as a 'probable carcinogen' because of its association with certain cancers, turn up in much of the food we eat, from tea to honey to oatmeal.[11] Glyphosate can also enter our bodies via our skin.

More recently, an Italian study found that long-term exposure to glyphosate affected the microbiome and hormones of rats.[12] If you're concerned, several laboratories now offer testing services for both glyphosate and other commonly used pesticides.

Cancer isn't the only disease linked to pesticides, however. A study from Duke University found that people exposed to pesticides were 42 per cent more likely to develop Alzheimer's, while researchers at the Banner Alzheimer's Institute in Arizona believe that toxic chemicals are more powerful than genes in triggering dementia.[13] Studies now suggest that exposure to pesticides at both high and low levels, particularly when over the long term, causes cellular damage that might lead to both cancer and neurological disorders.[14]

There's growing evidence of a link between exposure to pesticides (in particular two common agrochemicals called maneb and paraquat) and Parkinson's disease.[15] A recent study found those with a genetic predisposition to Parkinson's disease who were exposed to low levels of maneb or paraquat had a 250 per cent greater chance of developing the disease.[16] Meanwhile, other studies have linked pesticide exposure to diabetes.[17]

It's impossible to live in the modern world without some exposure to pesticides, but there are a few simple things we can do to minimise our risks:

- Eat organic/home-grown when you can: a US study of 4,500 people found that those who 'often or always' ate organic had 65 per cent fewer pesticide residues in their urine.[18]
- Grow your own, but without herbicides and insecticides.

- Invest in a water filtration system to reduce trace pesticides in your drinking water.

Doing the following will also help avoid unnecessary chemicals:

- Use environmentally friendly cleaning products.
- Use traps, baits and swatters to control vermin and insects rather than poison.
- Avoid unnecessary dry cleaning.
- Microwave using glass rather than plastic.
- Use deodorants rather than aluminium-containing antiperspirants.
- Choose organic cosmetics over chemical cosmetics (see our website for our favourite products).

If you've been exposed to high levels of pesticides for any length of time, ask your GP to refer you for testing (it's a simple urine test).

Clean out your medicine cabinet of anticholinergics

Clearing out the very cabinet that's supposed to keep you well might sound like back-to-front thinking, but it's exactly what we did. Most of us now take a pill for something, even if it's only an aspirin. But there's evidence that some of the pills we routinely pop (without a second thought) might be doing us more harm than good. These days, we ask ourselves: 'Do I need this and is there an alternative?' Never stop prescribed medication without checking with your GP first, obviously, but be aware that the spotlight, as we wrote this book, was on anticholinergics.

Found in several antidepressants, bladder drugs and medication for Parkinson's disease, anticholinergics block a nervous-system neurotransmitter called acetylcholine which helps to regulate some of the body's most basic functions, from bladder control and fine motor skills to thinking, motivation and memory. Research suggests that about 10 per cent of over fifties regularly take medication containing anticholinergics, although this figure could be much higher.[19]

Why do we need to know this? Because taking medication containing anticholinergics is thought to increase the risk of dementia. The first reports suggesting a possible link appeared almost a decade ago. Then, in 2015, a large American study[20] found a clear link between elderly people taking high levels of anticholinergics and the onset of Alzheimer's. But it wasn't until 2018 – and a much larger study – that the medical community sat up and took note.

In a study published in the *BMJ*,[21] researchers looked at the medical and prescription records of 325,000 over-sixty-fives and found that taking a strong anticholinergic for as little as a year lead to a 30 per cent increase in dementia risk. In some cases there was a 15–20-year gap between taking the medication and the onset of dementia. And the higher the dosage, the greater the risk – findings that mirrored those of several earlier studies. The drugs with the clearest associations were identified as: amitriptyline, dosulepin and paroxetine (in antidepressants); oxybutynin, solifenacin and tolterodine (for incontinence); and procyclidine (for Parkinson's Disease).

The report's authors urged GPs to think twice before routinely prescribing medication containing high levels of anticholinergics; however, not all such drugs are prescribed by GPs. Many are sold over the counter, although no link was found between dementia and the less potent anticholinergics found in antihistamines and travel sickness pills.

On a more positive note, the speculated association between proton pump inhibitors (PPIs, often used for acid-related gastrointestinal disorders like dyspepsia) and dementia has been temporarily laid to rest by a 2017 report that found no link.[22]

Whereas the Alzheimer's Society suggest anticholinergics shouldn't be prescribed to over-sixty-fives, we would go further:

- If you're using over-the-counter remedies and suspect that they might contain anticholinergics, check with your pharmacist.
- Ask yourself: 'Do I need this medication?' Many of the experts we spoke to suggested that people often take medication out of habit, even when it doesn't work.
- If you need the medication, can you change to a less potent form?
- Always check the anticholinergic content of any prescription you're given – and remember that if you're taking several meds each containing low doses of anticholinergic, you need to consider the *total* dosage.
- Never stop taking prescribed medication without consulting your doctor.

CHAPTER 14

Rethinking Ageing – Our Closing thoughts

Inspiration from SuperAgers

While we relish grappling with statistics and exploring the findings of so many remarkable researchers from across the world, reading scientific reports can resemble chewing on cardboard. Interviewing SuperAgers, however, was an unadulterated joy. Sadly, our book only has room for five, but each of the five nonagenarians profiled here is hugely inspirational. While all five are very different, they have several things in common: a distinct sense of purpose and intention; a manifest desire to be cheerfully alive; a history of eating home-cooked food; active lives that include walking, tennis and yoga (for example). In addition, they are all British – and subject to the vagaries of our climate – and they all live in their own homes, giving them a continued sense of independence. In every other way they are different. Some have close families, some have no families. One lives in the remote country, one lives in a northern city. Some had been heavy smokers, others had never touched a cigarette. Some have university educations, others left school at 14. And so on. Regardless of their similarities and differences, we hope you find them as inspirational as we do.

CASE STUDY

Helen Holder, 96

'Everyone wants something that is their own and is slightly creative.'

The story of Helen is one of the most inspiring we've come across. Although Helen's grandmother lived to 98, her father came from a short-lived family and died at 60. Helen wasn't expected to live beyond six months. For years she had poor health, regularly succumbing to respiratory and chest infections. 'I was never robust,' she says. 'I was frequently off work with something or other.'

Helen went to an academic school and recalls being 'hopeless at drawing and painting'. But she enjoyed visiting galleries, often alone and even in wartime. Her interest was greatly increased when she married an eminent picture dealer, although she never considered painting or drawing until after she retired. With time on her hands she signed up for an untutored art class. Later she joined another class, tutored by a local artist. She was 84 when her husband died, at which point she began working more purposefully at her art. 'I worked very hard,' she explains. 'It was a real slog, but the other artists were encouraging and I had a renewed sense of purpose.'

By the time Helen reached her ninetieth birthday, she'd been painting for 26 years. She invited a local gallery owner to see some of her work and, as she unveiled her paintings, the gallery owner's eyes lit up. 'I can see a wonderful exhibition,' she declared.

Helen had her first exhibition shortly after her ninetieth birthday. She sold every painting. She had a second exhibition at the age of 93 and, again, sold every picture.

Although Helen was a smoker into her fifties, she has always been a keen walker with a love of hill walking. She started a weekly yoga class in her forties but is best known in her local town for her paintings and her parties. 'I'm very gregarious,' she adds. 'People and painting give me purpose. Most importantly, we all want something that is our own and … creative.'

CASE STUDY

Douglas Matthews, 92

Douglas Matthews is an alert, thoughtful 92-year-old who still works seven days a week. Is it his work that keeps him young or his youthfulness that keeps him working?

Douglas has never taken a vitamin supplement, or embarked on an exercise regime. He's never followed a special diet, preferring traditional English food that he often cooks himself ('and always with greens'). But, without being aware of it, he's rigorously trained his brain. How has he done this? Part of the answer is: work.

When Douglas retired from his job as head librarian of the London Library, he began working as a freelance indexer, a job he intends to do for as long as he can.

'I work at least four hours every day, including weekends,' he says. 'If I'm on a tight deadline, I'll put in seven hours a day until the book is finished, often working until 11.30 at night.'

Douglas finds his work immensely rewarding. 'If I'm ever in between jobs I become a bit fretful. I need to work, not for financial reasons, but because it's what I do. Every time I finish indexing a book I feel a real sense of accomplishment. What else would give me this?'

This sense of purpose and accomplishment undoubtedly contributes to Douglas's superb ageing (see 'Find Your Sense of Purpose' on page 241). But there's another factor at play too. His work forces him to keep learning, to keep grappling with new ideas, new subject matter, new areas of history or geography or science. 'The books I index are often very challenging, so I always learn a huge amount. To produce a really good index you have to engage very deeply with the text. You can't skim or speed-read.' In the last year alone, Douglas has learnt about Napoleon, Charles Darwin, the Yangtze Valley and the history of the Jews, among other subjects.

Despite spending hours poring over the written word, Douglas reads every night for pleasure: 'I always read a book before I go to sleep, even if I've been indexing late into the night.' (See 'Why Do Book Readers Live Longer?' on page 229.) But it's not only reading and working that keep his brain growing. Douglas spends 30 minutes every day doing *The Times* cryptic crossword *in his head*. He refuses to write down the answers; instead, he forces himself to commit the entire crossword visually to memory. We now know that a habitual crossword done on autopilot does surprisingly little for the brain, but challenging oneself, as Douglas does, keeps the brain well exercised.

A lifetime of playing the piano might have helped, too. Douglas was learning new pieces of music into his eighties, in order to accompany his daughter, a professional singer.

'It's all quite sedentary,' he adds. 'I work in hourly chunks and try to walk as much as I can. I think everyone needs something purposeful and productive in their life: be it work or volunteering. A retirement of hobbies isn't enough.'

CASE STUDY

Lady Kenya Tatton-Brown, 96

Lady Kenya was named after Africa's second-highest mountain: Mount Kenya. It's a fitting name for someone who's aged as impressively and formidably as she has.

On the day we interviewed her – in the home she's lived in for over 50 years – she'd read *The Times*, dipped into the novel she was currently reading and read a few pages (in French) of a book on the architecture of Chartres Cathedral. She was also heading off on a 70-mile journey to hear a lecture on Anglo-American history.

How has Lady Kenya managed to preserve her vigour and vim? 'I come from a different generation,' she says. 'I joined the Royal Navy as a Wren and spent four years serving in the Second World War. It was a traumatising but formative experience that toughened me up and taught me that life isn't fair. When the War was over I decided to qualify as a physiotherapist. Most women of my background didn't work in those days, but I wanted to, even after I married and had children. I worked part-time and my wages paid for a nanny.'

When her husband died, Lady Kenya was only in her forties with three children to support. 'I set up a private physiotherapy practice in my house and never looked back.'

She worked as a physiotherapist all her life, giving up her final patient at the age of 91. The nature of her work gave her an excellent understanding of the physical body – its bones, muscles and ligaments. 'My top tip for anyone wanting to live to a good old age is to keep moving,' she explains. 'I grew up encouraged to take a walk every single day, whatever the weather, and I still do this. Walking was a pleasure not a chore.' For years Lady Kenya had dogs that needed twice-daily walks, but she also kept fit by riding, gardening and playing tennis – she played her last game of tennis on her ninetieth birthday.

'I can't play now, so I've devised an exercise routine that I do almost every day. I spend ten minutes moving every muscle group in my body, just small movements – a minute on each muscle group – as I lie in bed. It's vital to keep moving,' she says.

But Lady Kenya has done more than keep herself physically fit. She's kept herself mentally fit, too. In addition to her daily reading (her house was notably full of books), she immerses herself in family history, transcribing letters and diaries on her computer. 'I force myself to do the Code Words puzzle in the newspaper every day, and I try to read in French even though I'm rusty,' she adds.

Having faith is also important to Lady Kenya. She attended church every week until recently and sat on 'every church committee, from the sewing committee to being a church warden'.

She has always eaten classic English home-cooked food with seasonal vegetables. 'We were all taught to cook,' she says. 'As a girl, I spent six months at cookery school, so I've always cooked from scratch with whatever's fresh and available. I enjoy cooking, so I never bought a ready meal for my family. But I hated cleaning! I've barely wielded a hoover ... my earnings paid for a cleaner, but if the cleaner couldn't come I let the house get dirty. It never bothered me.'

For the last decade Lady Kenya has taken a multivitamin during the winter ('when I remember') but she's taken no other supplements, no special 'superfoods' and has never followed a diet. When we interviewed her she was organising a hog roast for her forthcoming birthday party.

'You've got to keep moving,' she stresses. 'Keep moving – keep thinking and having opinions.' She points at *The Times* and adds, 'This article made me want to write a letter to the editor ...'

CASE STUDY

Margaret Hibbert, 96

Margaret has seven grandchildren, eight great-grandchildren and three great-great-grandchildren. During her long life she's experienced many setbacks, from a tumour that necessitated a full hysterectomy in her forties, to carpal tunnel syndrome in both hands, to being hit by a lorry at the age of 92. And yet, Margaret, who still lives alone, remains as sharp and bright-eyed as someone half her age, so what's her secret?

In spite of being a single mother of five, Margaret had a frenzied career as a private investigator, attending courts and trials not only across the UK but across the world. She loved her work (only retiring at 70 after a slipped disc resulted in a laminectomy), but described it as '24/7, with no time for leisure and no regular hours for eating or sleeping or exercise, as I was always on call.'

But she always cooked meals for her family and rarely resorted to ready meals. 'Meat or fish with vegetables and always a desert, my children loved apple pie and rhubarb and custard although I'm more of a savoury person,' she explains. 'Our food was traditional English food: rib of beef with Yorkshire pudding or chicken with home-made stuffing, although I've never eaten meat on Fridays.' Margaret's father was a gardener on a large estate and she grew up with a constant supply of seasonal fresh fruit and vegetables. 'Until quite recently I bottled fruit and vegetables in season, as my mother did, but I can't buy shop fruit as it doesn't taste right to me, not like the fruit I grew up with.'

No doubt a childhood spent eating organic fruit and vegetables straight from the garden has aided Margaret's longevity. But her siblings (one of whom was Annabel's grandmother) died a long time ago, suggesting something else is at play. Like our other Age-Well inspirations, Margaret has a powerful sense of purpose (see Chapter 10). After retiring she became very involved in caring for the less fortunate, visiting the bereaved, the sick and the lonely. 'I attended courses at several local hospices and worked for 25 years as a volunteer for the St Vincent de Paul Society, a faith-driven charity tackling poverty and loneliness. I still do what I can by phone or letter.' (See 'Sharing, Caring, Community and Humanity Matter' on page 207.)

Her purpose and altruism are driven by her deeply rooted faith. Research has shown that faith can play a vital role in longevity, something reflected in the world's Blue Zones. Margaret is the living embodiment of this. 'I always go to mass on Sundays and Holy Days,' she says. 'I went every day after I retired, and now I watch the daily service on the Internet. I'd find it very hard to carry on without having faith in my life.' Margaret prays for a few minutes every morning and every evening, 'to give thanks for just being here – I have so much for which to give thanks'.

Margaret's faith provides her with a community, a sense of purpose and gratitude, and a serenity that keeps the future bright with hope. 'I'm looking forward to a life hereafter. I don't know what form it'll take, but I'm excited at the prospect of finding out. Our bodies are too wonderful to simply end. I believe life is eternal and will be an adventure for us all.'

CASE STUDY

Sam Almond, 92

Sam Almond is the UK's champion swimmer in the 90–95 age category. Now 92, he swims five mornings a week, a habit he hopes to continue as long as he can.

'Our body is the most important thing we have, more important than our house or our car,' he explains over a large glass of water at his local gym. 'I'm in the pool by 6.30am and I swim for a good 12 minutes: backstroke, breaststroke and front crawl. Until recently, I swam in the sea every morning between May and September, and was always on the beach by 6.00am. Swimming is a habit now, like cleaning my teeth.'

Throughout his seventies and eighties, Sam also walked and cycled every day, but foot problems limit him to swimming now. 'Swimming is brilliant because it puts no pressure on my joints,' he adds.

Before Sam swims, he drinks a pint of water and spends 15 minutes stretching each of his muscles, a series of movements he devised after reading several books on longevity. 'My stretching routine helps with my sense of balance. As I got older, I felt my balance going, but this routine has improved it enormously.'

Sam wasn't always as healthy as he is now. 'Until my mid-forties I smoked 70 cigarettes a day. Then I heard someone on the radio explaining how dangerous smoking was. I stopped smoking that very day. We all need to prepare for our retirement years. It's about self-discipline and habit. Now I snack on nuts and drink beetroot juice.'

In order to prepare for the last third of his life, Sam read every book he could find and then wrote his own longevity guide which he self-published (see Bibliography). 'Excluding family, exercise is the most important thing,' he says. 'We also need to avoid processed food and stay interested in life. I'm a keen private investor and follow the money markets every day. It helps me stay focused and engaged.'

Sam also attributes his mental agility to his wife, Hazel.

'We compete over the word puzzles in the newspaper; we argue, we exchange banter, we tease each other.'

Sam's final tip is a daily nap. 'Every afternoon I put on my pyjamas and sleep for at least an hour, sometimes three hours. I've been napping since I retired at 65, and I recommend it to anyone wanting a long and healthy life.'

... and finally

Once we reach 40 we can no longer take our future health for granted. As Professor Hornberger says, 'Dementia is a disease of middle age presenting in old age, but 30 per cent of all cases are preventable which is why we need to make lifestyle changes as early as possible.'[1] From middle age onwards (and ideally before) we need to nurture our bodies and brains; we need to give our health the priority it deserves; we need to treat our future well-being as a project.

We hope this book has inspired you to start your own Age-Well Project. Over the last five years we've learnt many things, but the most important has been this: taking control of your health is supremely liberating. We never aimed for perfection, just progression – one step at a time.

We never followed prescriptive diets, draconian exercise regimes or costly supplement programmes. Instead we made time to cook, dance, hike through forests, experiment with herbs and spices, play ping-pong, meditate, fill our houses with greenery, and floss our teeth! We overhauled our larders (no more junk food) and restructured our days to include longer overnight fasts, fewer lie-ins and time for cooking and exercise. But we did it slowly and, on the occasions we fell off the Age-Well wagon (and it will happen), we read, blogged and helped each other back, guilt-free. Which is a good reason to embark on your own project with a friend or family member.

Our lifestyle changes worked: we feel better in our fifties than we've ever felt. We have more energy, we sleep better, feel happier and have fewer ailments than we had in our youth. We'd love you to feel as good, whatever your age.

Equally importantly, we hope this book has encouraged you to think *beyond* yourself – to family, friends, community and society. We'd like to see our Age-Well Project reach as many people as possible. By being healthy ourselves, and encouraging others to do the same, we make the world a more hopeful and humane place.

For the health and happiness of our elderly to be fully realised we also need a reappraisal of the role of older people in society. Some of the most poignant studies we've uncovered have been those showing how older people flourish in communities where they are respected and celebrated. As well as tackling your own health, we'd love you to think more broadly about how we recreate a society in which the elderly are treated with the inclusion and dignity they deserve.

It's time to reframe our notion of ageing. Growing older, done with consciousness and care, is not something to be denied, feared or repelled by. Rather, it's a new chapter in life, one that brings its own joys and challenges. Understand it, welcome it, enjoy the good bits and reframe the bad bits. Develop your grit!

This is not the end of our Age-Well Project. In many ways the medical community is only just beginning to understand how our bodies work, how they interact with both the natural and man-made environments in which we live. This is the golden age of medical science: as researchers continue to unpick the complex inter-relationship of genes, cells, phytonutrients, bio-chemicals, microbiota, neurons (and so on), we expect more and more studies on how best to fend off the diseases of ageing. But there's one thing we're fairly certain of: there'll be no magic pill, no elixir of youth. Our prediction is that lifestyle changes will continue to dominate the Age-Well agenda. Stay with us at agewellproject.com.

Age is just a number.

The rest is up to you.

CHAPTER 15

Recipes

The Age-Well Vegetable Sauté

Our age-well sauté technique is a traditional Chinese cooking method, involving a scrape of fat, followed by a splash of water. This reduces the temperature of the oil, which, in turn, reduces the production of aldehydes and free radicals.

We use this for all kinds of vegetables, but try to include some greens, a prebiotic allium such as leek or onion and something chunkier like mushrooms or peppers. We serve this with fish, meat, a poached egg or simply over a bowl of grains. Use the recipe below as guidance rather than scripture.

Serves 2–3
30g walnuts, pumpkin seeds or pine nuts
1 tbsp coconut oil or light olive oil
150g mushrooms, sliced
2 small or 1 large leek, sliced
½ red pepper, deseeded and chopped

1 garlic clove, crushed

1 tsp dried oregano or thyme

½ tsp ground turmeric

1 tsp ginger paste, or 1cm fresh root ginger, peeled and
   finely grated

2 handfuls of spring greens or kale, chopped

salt and ground black pepper

Toast the walnuts or seeds in a dry pan over a medium heat until they darken and start to smell nutty. Leave to one side.

Keep a small jug of water beside the hob as you cook. Heat a large frying pan over a medium-high heat. Add the oil and reduce the temperature to medium. Add the mushrooms, leeks and pepper, and cook for 5 minutes or until they start to soften. Add water if they start to stick.

Add the garlic, oregano and spices, and cook for 30 seconds. Add the greens or kale and a good splash of water. Keep stirring and cooking for 1–2 minutes, adding a drop more water if necessary, then cover and cook for another 2 minutes. Give it all a final stir, season well with salt and pepper and sprinkle over the nuts or seeds. Serve.

Nacho Soup

This flavoursome, hearty soup contains two types of beans and is packed with plant protein and fibre. It also gets a big thumbs up from our children!

Serves 4

1 tbsp olive oil

1 onion, finely chopped

2 garlic cloves, finely chopped

2 tsp ground cumin

1 tsp sweet smoked paprika

1 tsp chilli powder, plus more to taste

1 tsp ground cinnamon

400g tin red kidney beans, drained and rinsed

400g tin black beans, drained and rinsed

100g sweetcorn kernels (no need to defrost if frozen)

500ml vegetable stock

500g passata

100g tomato salsa (from a jar or tub)

salt and ground black pepper

To finish:

2 tbsp chopped fresh coriander

2 handfuls of lightly salted tortilla chips (optional)

1 ripe avocado, halved, peeled and diced

1 lime, quartered, to serve

Heat the oil in a large saucepan over a medium heat and cook the onion for 5 minutes or until translucent but not browned. Add the garlic and spices, and cook for another 30 seconds. Add the remaining soup ingredients. Bring to the boil, cover and simmer gently for 20 minutes.

Transfer three ladlefuls of the soup to a blender or food processor and blend until smooth. Return the purée to the pan, mix well and reheat. Season well to taste, adding more chilli if that's your thing.

Serve the soup topped with fresh coriander, tortilla chips (if using) and avocado, with a lime quarter to squeeze over.

Simple Yoghurt Sauce

This simple sauce is made in seconds and can be dolloped onto anything, dropped into a simple vegetable soup, or used as a dip. Full of probiotics, we like it with plain grilled fish or smeared thickly over steamed vegetables for a light lunch. To increase or alter the probiotic content, use kefir-style yoghurt or sheep's yoghurt, which often carry additional strains. We use ready-made chermoula (North African spice paste) or zhoug (Yemenite spice paste), both of which can be found in some supermarkets, online or in Middle-Eastern shops.

Serves 4
4 tbsp yoghurt (the creamier the better)
1 tbsp chermoula or zhoug paste

Mix until blended and serve as an accompaniment to ... just about anything.

Peanut Noodles

This rich, satisfying dish makes a speedy week-night dinner and can easily be adapted for meat-eaters or vegans. Both versions benefit from the nutrient-rich properties of nuts and spinach.

Serves 4
1 tbsp olive oil
400g minced turkey or drained, crumbled tofu
300g noodles, such as buckwheat
2 garlic cloves, crushed

1 tsp ginger paste or 1cm fresh root ginger, peeled and
    finely grated
200g spinach
2 tbsp unsalted peanuts, chopped

For the sauce:
4 tbsp smooth peanut butter
2 tbsp reduced-salt soy sauce
2 tbsp rice vinegar
½ tbsp maple syrup
a pinch of chilli flakes or powder, or to taste

To make the sauce, put the sauce ingredients in a bowl and add 100ml warm water. Whisk together to combine well. Taste to check the balance of acid, sweet and salt, adjust as necessary, then leave to one side.

Heat the oil in a large frying pan over a medium heat. Turn the heat up to high and add the turkey or tofu. Fry for 5 minutes, without moving it around too much, so that it starts to brown and crisp. Meanwhile, cook the noodles in a saucepan of boiling water for 3 minutes, or according to the pack instructions. Drain in a colander.

Reduce the heat under the frying pan, then add the garlic, ginger and spinach. Stir-fry for 2 minutes. Add the noodles and drizzle over the sauce, adding a splash of water if needed. Toss around in the pan until it's piping hot, then sprinkle over the chopped peanuts and serve immediately.

Massaged Kabbouleh

This version of the Middle Eastern classic tabbouleh replaces the traditional parsley with kale (kale + tabbouleh = kabbouleh!). Don't be afraid to get your hands messy – massaging the kale improves its flavour and texture, so it's softer and less 'raw'.

Serves 4 as a side dish
30g quinoa, well rinsed
2 tbsp raisins or sultanas
2 tbsp apple cider vinegar
30g walnuts
200g kale, tough stalks removed, leaves chopped
1 tbsp olive oil
½ tsp salt
¼ cucumber, quartered lengthways and chopped
2 tbsp chopped fresh parsley

Put the quinoa in a saucepan and add double the volume of boiling water. Bring to the boil, then simmer for 15 minutes or until tender, or according to the pack instructions. Drain in a sieve and leave to cool. Put the dried fruit in a bowl and add the vinegar. Leave to soak while you prepare the other ingredients.

Toast the walnuts in a dry pan over a medium heat until they darken and start to smell nutty. Leave to one side.

Put the kale in a large bowl. Add the olive oil and salt, and massage for 2 minutes or until the kale starts to wilt and collapse. Add the remaining ingredients, the quinoa, fruit and nuts. If you have time, leave to stand for 20 minutes so the flavours meld.

Sweet Potato Supper Bowl

A vegetarian meal in a bowl – sweet, warming and delicious. The trick is to start the sweet potato slices in a cold oven, allowing the sugars to caramelise as they slowly heat up.

Serves 4

2 tbsp olive oil, plus extra for greasing

4 sweet potatoes (about 750g), cut into 5mm slices – no need to peel but do if you prefer

1 small red onion, sliced

1 garlic clove, crushed

½ tsp ground turmeric

1 tsp ground cumin

1 tsp sweet smoked paprika

200g kale, tough stalks removed, leaves chopped

1 tbsp red wine vinegar

4 eggs

40g salted cashew nuts, chopped

chilli sauce

Lightly oil two baking sheets. Lay the sweet potato slices on the baking sheets, making sure they don't overlap, then cover tightly with foil. Put the baking sheets into a cold oven and set the temperature to 180°C (160°C fan oven), Gas 4. Cook for 30 minutes, then carefully remove the foil. Return the sweet potatoes to the oven for another 10 minutes. You should have delicious soft, caramelised sweet potato.

While the sweet potato is cooking, heat 1 tbsp of the olive oil in a large frying pan. Cook the onion until soft. Add the garlic and spices and cook for 30 seconds. Add the kale to the pan with a splash of water. Cook until the kale is just wilted, then stir in the vinegar.

Take the kale mixture out of the pan and keep warm while you heat the remaining oil. Fry the eggs until cooked to your liking. Arrange the sweet potato slices in individual bowls and top with the kale mix. Put an egg on each and add a sprinkling of cashew nuts. Serve with chilli sauce.

Warm Roasted Vegetables with Pomegranate Two Ways

We love pomegranates, both for their immune-supporting properties and for their sweet and sour flavour. This is a meal-in-a-tray: everything goes in the oven in one roasting dish, add a few toppings, and dinner is served.

Serves 4

2 tbsp olive oil

1 tbsp pomegranate molasses, plus extra to serve

350g peeled butternut squash, or other winter squash, and/or
   sweet potatoes, cut into slices

3 red and/or orange peppers, deseeded and chopped

400g tin chickpeas, drained and rinsed

100g baby spinach leaves

100g ricotta

2 tbsp chopped fresh mint

2 tbsp pomegranate seeds

salt and ground black pepper

Preheat the oven to 180°C (160°C fan oven), Gas 4. In a bowl, mix the oil and pomegranate molasses. Season well with salt and pepper. Put the squash, peppers and chickpeas in a large roasting tin. Pour over the oil mixture and mix well (we use our hands to massage it into the vegetables). Roast for 30 minutes, or until the vegetables are very soft and starting to brown at the edges.

Take out of the oven and stir in the spinach. Tip the whole lot into a serving bowl and dollop over teaspoonfuls of the ricotta, mint and pomegranate seeds. Drizzle over a little more molasses just before serving.

Age-Well Salsa Verde

As we've added more whole grains and vegetables to our diets we've sensed a need for punchy, flavour-packed sauces. Every ingredient in this salsa is an age-well booster: olive oil, oily fish, walnuts, herbs ... the list goes on.

Serves 4 as a condiment
1 garlic clove, peeled
10g each of fresh basil, flat-leaf parsley and mint, tough
    stems removed
1 tbsp capers, rinsed
3 anchovy fillets in oil
30g walnuts
1 tbsp Dijon mustard
1 tbsp apple cider vinegar
6 tbsp good olive oil
salt and ground black pepper

You can make this in a blender, but the results are much better when you chop by hand. Finely chop the garlic on a large chopping board. Add the herbs and keep chopping. When they're all finely chopped, add the capers, anchovies and walnuts, and keep chopping. When you're happy with the texture, scoop everything into a bowl. Stir in the mustard, vinegar and oil. Stir well and season to taste with salt and pepper. Serve.

Vegetable Chickpea Pancakes

These chunky pancakes make use of chickpea flour (also known as gram flour), which is gluten-free and high in protein. You'll find it in Asian or health food shops.

Serves 4

2 carrots

1 courgette

4 eggs

2 tbsp chopped fresh herbs, such as mint and/or coriander

1 garlic clove, finely chopped

1 tsp ground coriander

1 tsp ground cumin

½ tsp ground turmeric

75g chickpea (gram) flour

light olive oil, for shallow frying

salt and ground black pepper

4 tbsp Greek yoghurt, to serve

Grate the carrots and courgette together. Put in a sieve with a couple of large pinches of salt and leave to drain for 10 minutes or so. (If you're really pushed for time, skip this step. The end result may be a little more moist and you'll need to add salt later.)

Beat the eggs in a large bowl, add the herbs, garlic, spices and chickpea flour. Season with pepper (and salt if you haven't salted the vegetables earlier). Whisk together. Squeeze the vegetables to expel any liquid, then add to the egg mixture.

Heat a frying pan over a medium-high heat and add a little oil. Add four heaped tablespoons of the vegetable mixture to the pan to make four large pancakes. Cook until the underside is brown, then flip over. Reduce the heat to allow them to cook through. Repeat until you've used up all the mixture. Serve with a dollop of yoghurt.

Age-Well Poke Bowl

Poke (pronounced pok-ah) is an Hawaiian dish, essentially deconstructed sushi with lots of delicious additions. It's very versatile: you can experiment with the vegetables and toppings, but always use the freshest raw fish you can find.

Serves 4
400g best salmon, skinned and diced into 1cm cubes
100g brown rice, well rinsed
150g edamame beans, cooked
50g cashew nuts
50g chopped kale leaves (without stalks) or baby
   spinach leaves
2 carrots, grated
¼ red cabbage, thinly sliced
100g pineapple flesh, cubed

For the dressing:
1 tsp ginger paste or 1cm fresh root ginger, peeled and
   finely grated
1 tsp chilli sauce

1 tbsp lemon juice

2 tbsp sesame oil

2 tbsp reduced-salt soy sauce

2 tbsp rice vinegar

To make the dressing, put all the dressing ingredients in a bowl and whisk together. Put the salmon in a shallow dish and pour over half the dressing. Mix well, then leave to marinate while you assemble the other ingredients.

Put the rice in a saucepan and add double the volume of boiling water. Bring to the boil, then simmer for 25 minutes or until tender, or according to the pack instructions. Drain in a sieve and leave to cool.

Meanwhile, cook the edamame beans in a saucepan of boiling water for 5 minutes or according to the pack instructions. Drain in a colander.

Toast the cashew nuts in a dry pan over a medium heat until golden and they start to smell nutty. Chop finely, then leave to one side.

Divide the rice among four serving bowls and top with the raw kale or spinach. Put the prepared vegetables, pineapple and cashew nuts on top of the rice and leaf base, so that you get lots of bursts of colour. Add the salmon and drizzle over the remaining dressing. Serve.

Braised Beef with Quinoa and Lentils

We eat far less red meat now so, when we do, we want hearty, satisfying dishes. This hits the spot. Buy the best quality beef you can afford, preferably organic.

Serves 4

800g piece of beef brisket

1 tbsp olive oil

2 carrots, roughly chopped

1 onion, roughly chopped

4 mushrooms, quartered

3 garlic cloves, unpeeled

2 bay leaves

1 thyme sprig

250ml red wine

250ml beef stock

100g quinoa, well rinsed

150g cooked Puy lentils, drained

150g baby spinach

salt and ground black pepper

creamed horseradish, to serve

Preheat the oven to 170°C (150°C fan oven), Gas 3. Season the meat well with salt and pepper. Heat the oil in a flameproof casserole and sear the meat so that it starts to brown. Remove from the pan and put on a plate.

Sauté the carrots, onion and mushrooms in the fat that remains in the casserole for 5 minutes. Add the garlic, herbs, beef, wine and stock. Bring to the boil, then cover and transfer to the oven for 2½ hours, turning the beef over half-way through.

Carefully lift the beef and vegetables out of the cooking liquid, and put them on a plate. Cover with foil and leave to rest. Take out the herbs and discard them. Take out the garlic and squeeze the pulp back into the pan. Add the quinoa to the liquid remaining in the pan, bring to the boil and simmer for 10 minutes or until the quinoa is cooked through. Stir in the lentils and spinach, and heat through.

Divide the lentil mixture between warm serving bowls and top with slices of beef and the braised vegetables. A dollop of horseradish is great with this dish.

Persian Chickpea and Walnut Stew

This satisfying stew has all the heartiness of meat, but is, in fact, vegan. The ground walnuts add thickness and plenty of healthy fats.

Serves 4
100g walnuts
1 tbsp olive oil
1 large onion, finely sliced
1 garlic clove, finely chopped
½ tsp ground turmeric
½ tsp ground cinnamon
500g mushrooms, quartered
400g tin chickpeas, undrained
100ml pomegranate molasses
salt and ground black pepper
1 tbsp chopped fresh mint leaves and 1 tbsp fresh
    pomegranate seeds, to garnish
rice, to serve

Toast the walnuts in a dry pan over a medium heat until they darken and start to smell nutty. Leave to cool slightly, then blitz in a food processor until they are finely ground, being careful not to let the mixture turn into walnut butter.

Heat the oil in a saucepan over a low heat and cook the onions for 10 minutes or until very soft and starting to brown. Add the garlic and spices, and cook for 30 seconds. Add the mushrooms and allow to cook for 5 minutes, stirring frequently until they start to shrink and release liquid. Add the chickpeas and their liquid, the ground walnuts and the pomegranate molasses. Season well with salt and pepper, and simmer for 15 minutes until thickened. Serve with rice, garnished with the mint and a sprinkling of pomegranate seeds.

Carrot-Top Pesto

This is the perfect way to use up the carrot tops and fronds that otherwise go to waste. Our children prefer it to normal basil pesto and hoover it up with carrot batons or crackers. Otherwise, use it as you'd use any pesto: on fish, pasta, grains or vegetables.

70g carrot tops, stalks and all
2 garlic cloves, peeled and left whole
7 tbsp extra virgin olive oil
2 tbsp cashew nuts, or pine nuts, or any nut you like
a large palmful of freshly grated Parmesan cheese
a pinch of salt

Wash and dry the carrot tops (if they need it), then put everything in a blender or food processor and blitz for 30 seconds.

Banana and Wheatgerm Loaf

It took weeks of experimenting to devise the perfect afternoon cake. Our children eventually chose this as their absolute favourite, preferably eaten warm straight from the oven. You can replace the sultanas with walnuts for the sake of variety (in which case they don't need soaking).

> 1 cup of black or ginger tea (made from a tea bag)
> 100g sultanas
> 150g wholemeal self-raising flour
> 25g wheatgerm
> 1 tsp cinnamon
> 100g butter
> 150g honey or maple syrup
> 1 tsp vanilla extract
> 2 eggs, beaten
> 4 bananas, mashed

An hour or so before you plan to make the cake, brew a cup of hot tea (any tea you like; we are partial to ginger), add the sultanas and leave to soak. Alternatively simmer for a few minutes in a pan. You want the sultanas to be fat and juicy.

Heat the oven to 170°C (150°C fan oven), Gas 3. Grease and line a 23 × 12 cm loaf tin.

Mix the flour, wheatgerm and cinnamon in a bowl and set aside.

Melt the butter and honey over a low heat and stir until blended. Pour onto the dry ingredients. Add the vanilla extract, beaten eggs, mashed bananas and drained sultanas and stir well to combine.

Scrape everything into the loaf tin and bake for an hour or until an inserted skewer comes out clean. Leave to cool for 5 minutes, then turn out onto a wire rack.

Herby Za'atar Nuts

These nuts make the perfect pre-dinner nibble. The za'atar must include oregano and/or marjoram, two of the most antioxidant-rich herbs on the planet. We sometimes add an extra teaspoon of dried marjoram. Feel free to follow suit ...

Serves 10+
100g cashew nuts
100g walnuts
100g almonds
1½ tbsp olive oil
5 tsp za'atar mix
1 tsp good-quality salt (we like pink Himalayan mountain salt
   for this recipe)

Preheat the oven to 180°C (160°C fan oven), Gas 4. In a bowl, mix the nuts, oil, za'atar mix and salt, then spread them out in a roasting tin.

Bake for 12 minutes. They should be a pale golden-brown. Leave to cool before serving.

Double Sweetcorn Salad with Jalapeño and Lime Dressing

In this recipe, the mix of raw and cooked sweetcorn, alongside yellow peppers, provides a big dose of lutein to boost eye health. It's the perfect side dish for grilled chicken or barbecues.

Serves 4 as a side dish
2 yellow peppers, left whole
3 corn on the cobs

1 tbsp of jalapeño peppers (from a jar), finely chopped

1 tbsp brine from the jalapeño jar

juice of ½ lime

2 tbsp olive oil

1 tbsp chopped fresh coriander

Grill or barbecue the yellow peppers until the skins blacken and blister. Put them in a heatproof bowl and cover with clingfilm. Leave to one side to cool and allow the skins to steam off.

Meanwhile, grill or barbecue two of the corn cobs until they start to brown in patches. Leave them to cool, then stand a cob on one end on a chopping board. Run a sharp knife down the sides of the cob to release the kernels. Repeat with the other two cobs, so that you have a mixture of cooked and raw corn. Put into a serving bowl.

When the peppers are cool enough to handle, rub off the skins, remove and discard the seeds and stalk, and slice the flesh. Put in the serving bowl with the corn, and any juice that has collected in the bowl with the peppers.

Put the jalapeños in a small bowl and add the brine, lime juice and olive oil. Mix well together, then pour this over the corn and peppers. Stir, then top with the coriander and serve.

References

In the process of writing this book we consulted numerous sources of information (mostly academic research papers). These sources are acknowledged with a number in the relevant place in the text, enabling readers to delve deeper where required. In order to save paper (there are over 500 cited sources running to twenty-eight pages) we have placed the corresponding details of the citations on our website at agewellproject.com/book/references

References

Bibliography

While we relied primarily on research papers and studies, the following books were particularly helpful or inspiring and we have no hesitation in recommending them. Indeed, we urge you to read widely and to stay abreast of studies via some of the websites listed below.

The Telomere Effect, Elizabeth Blackburn and Elissa Epel (Orion Spring, 2017)

Younger: The Breakthrough Programme to Reset our Genes and Reverse Ageing, Sara Gottfried (Vermillion, 2017)

The Longevity Project, Howard S. Friedman and Leslie R. Martin (Hay House, 2011)

Why We Sleep, Matthew Walker (Allen Lane, 2017)

How to Sleep Well, Dr Neil Stanley, (Capstone, 2018)

The Longevity Diet, Dr Valter Longo (Penguin, 2018)

The Longevity Prescription, Robert Butler (Penguin, 2011)

The Longevity Bible, Cameron Diaz and Sandra Bark (Harper Wave, 2017)

How Not to Die, Michael Gregor (Pan, 2017)

Live Well to 101, Dawn Harper (Headline Home, 2018)

Dirty Genes: A Breakthrough Programme to Treat the Root Cause of Illness, Dr Ben Lynch (HarperOne, 2018)

Understanding Genetics, David Sadava (The Great Courses, 2008)

Healthy at 100, John Robbins (Ballantine Books, 2007)

The Clever Guts Diet, Michael Mosley (Short Books, 2017)

This Is Not a Diet Book, Bee Wilson (Fourth Estate, 2016)

100 Simple Things You Can Do to Prevent Alzheimer's, Jean Carper (Vermillion, 2011)

Brain Myths Exploded, Indre Viskontas (The Great Courses, 2017)

The Nature Fix, Florence Williams (W. W. Norton, 2018)

The Aging Brain, Professor Thad Polik (The Great Courses, 2016)

Nutrition Made Clear, Professor Roberta H. Anding (The Great Courses, 2013)

Genius Foods, Max Lugavere with Paul Grewal (Harper Wave, 2018)

Brain Rules for Aging Well, John Medina (Pear Press, 2017)

How God Changes Your Brain, Andrew Newberg and Mark Robert Waldman (Ballantine Books, 2010)

The Case Against Sugar, Gary Taubes (Portobello Books, 2018)

The 8-Week Blood Sugar Diet, Dr Michael Mosley (Short Books, 2015)

It Must Be My Hormones, Dr Marion Gluck and Vicki Edgson (Michael Joseph, 2017)

The Big Fat Surprise, Nina Teicholz (Scribe UK, 2015)

The End of Alzheimer's, Dr Dale Bredesen (Vermillion, 2017)

Grain Brain, Dr David Perlmutter (Yellow Kite, 2014)

The Alzheimer's Solution, Dr Dean Sherzai and Dr Ayesha Sherzai (Simon & Schuster UK, 2017)

The 4 Pillar Plan, Dr Rangan Chatterjee (Penguin Life, 2017)

Brain Food, Dr Lisa Mosconi (Penguin Life, 2018)

The China Study, T. Colin Campbell and Thomas M. Campbell II (BenBella Books, 2017)

Younger Next Year for Women, Chris Crowley and Henry S. Lodge (Workman Publishing, 2008)

Be Good to Your Gut, Eve Kalinik (Piatkus, 2017)

The Doctor's Kitchen, Dr Rupy Aujla (Harper Thorsons, 2017)

Websites

www.medicalnewstoday.com

www.pubmed.com

www.sciencedaily.com

www.sciencemag.org

https://joshmitteldorf.scienceblog.com

https://www.beingpatient.com/

www.bluezones.com

https://drmalcolmkendrick.org

We have also been inspired, over and over, by some marvellous cookery books. Far too many to list in their entirety, but the following are a few of our favourites:

Feasts, Sabrina Ghayour (Mitchell Beazley, 2017)

Persiana, Sabrina Ghayour (Mitchell Beazley, 2014)

The Middle Eastern Vegetarian Cookbook, Salma Hage (Phaidon Press, 2016)

Elly Pear's Let's Eat, Elly Curshen (Harper Thorsons, 2017)

The Flavour Thesaurus, Niki Segnit (Bloomsbury, 2010)

My Petite Kitchen, Eleonor Ozich (Murdoch Books, 2014)

How To Eat a Peach, Diana Henry (Mitchell Beazley, 2018)

A Change of Appetite, Diana Henry (Mitchell Beazley, 2014)

Radiant, Hanna Sillitoe (Kyle Books, 2017)

A Modern Way to Cook, Anna Jones (Fourth Estate, 2015)

A Modern Way to Eat, Anna Jones (Fourth Estate, 2014)

Dining In, Alison Roman (Clarkson Potter, 2017)

Super Natural Every Day, Heidi Swanson (Hardie Grant Books, 2017)

Plant-Powered Families, Dreena Burton (BenBella Books, 2015)

Index